POWER OF THIN

Change Your *Thinking*
Change Your *Weight*

Steve G. Jones & Frank Mangano

NEW YORK

POWER OF THIN

Change Your *Thinking*, Change Your *Weight*

Steve G. Jones & Frank Mangano

ISBN 978-1-61448-158-4 Paperback
ISBN 978-1-61448-159-1 eBook
Library of Congress Control Number: 2011940607

Published by:
MORGAN JAMES PUBLISHING
The Entrepreneurial Publisher
5 Penn Plaza, 23rd Floor
New York City, New York 10001
(212) 655-5470 Office
(516) 908-4496 Fax
www.MorganJamesPublishing.com

Cover Design by:
Rachel Lopez
rachel@r2cdesign.com

Interior Design by:
Bonnie Bushman
bbushman@bresnan.net

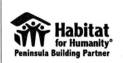

In an effort to support local communities, raise awareness and funds, Morgan James Publishing donates one percent of all book sales for the life of each book to Habitat for Humanity.
Get involved today, visit
www.HelpHabitatForHumanity.org.

MEDICAL DISCLAIMER

The information within this book is intended as reference material only, and not as medical or professional advice. Information contained herein is intended to give you the tools to make informed decisions about your lifestyle and health. It should not be used as a substitute for any treatment that has been prescribed or recommended by your doctor.

If you are currently taking medication for the treatment of obesity, continue to do so unless advised by your doctor to do otherwise. The author and publisher are not healthcare professionals, and expressly disclaim any responsibility for any adverse effects occurring as a result of the use of suggestions or information herein.

This book is offered as current information available about weight management, for your own education and enjoyment. If you have been told by a healthcare professional that you are overweight, then it is imperative that you seek the advice of your healthcare provider.

As always, never begin a dietary or exercise program without first consulting a qualified healthcare professional.

TABLE OF CONTENTS

Part Three Healthy Recipes   159

Part One

THE LAW OF ATTRACTION, HYPNOSIS AND WEIGHT LOSS

Chapter 1

INTRODUCTION

"Change in all things is sweet." —Aristotle

Everywhere we look it seems that people are struggling to lose weight. We see countless diet plans, diet course, pills, supplements, classes, and the list goes on... People are spending millions of dollars on weight loss products and services, and still not losing weight. Or, perhaps, even worse, they are losing some weight, but then gaining it all back weeks later.

According to the CDC, in the United States there has been a dramatic increase in obesity in the last 20 years. In fact, statistics compiled in 2008 showed that over 30 states had 20% or more of its population at the level of weight considered obese. In fact, in six states, more than 30% of people are obese. In case you were wondering, these states are Alabama, Mississippi, Oklahoma, South Carolina, Tennessee and West Virginia. According to more recent data published in the study "F as in Fat, How Obesity Policies are Failing in America 2009," the adult obesity rates have increased in 23 states just last year. No states report decreasing levels of obesity. This report also declared that more than 30 states have 30% of more obese children.

Obviously, losing weight is quite the struggle. Or is it? Here is an interesting idea to consider. Just because everyone is running around saying that it is difficult to lose weight, do we really know this is true? Do we know this beyond a shadow of a doubt? What if there was an easy solution that allowed the pounds to instantly melt away. It would be almost like magic. Is this a fantasy or is there a way to access this sort of magic? After all, we are adults. Shouldn't we have left these fairy tales behind us at this point in our lives?

As this book will show you, there is indeed a "magic bullet" that will allow you to lose weight. And it isn't complete fantasy either. In order to reach the diet goals you are seeking to reach, you only need to shift your thinking and follow certain easy guidelines. You just need to be willing to make changes in your thinking. Yes, the primary changes we are asking you to make aren't to go through every day starving and eating only carrot sticks. Nor are we asking you to go to the gym every night after work and work yourself into a frenzy sweating buckets. We will guide you through the dropping pounds through an easy process.

Through this book, we will guide you through the ideas of using the law of attraction and hypnosis to achieve a new level of health. This means that you will be able to be as thin as you want to be. Do you have clothes you have had sitting around that you haven't been able to wear for decades? If you want to wear them after following our guidelines, you will be able to do so. You will also be able to reach a new radiant level of health. This means that your body will feel revitalized, energetic and packed with energy.

And through this entire process, you will not feel as though you have to suffer. This means that you won't have the torment of struggling at the refrigerator over whether or not to eat that last piece of cheesecake. You will be able to go to any restaurant you choose, order what you want, and still not gain weight. Does this all sound too good to be true? If you read this book and follow the guidelines, you will find that indeed this all can occur for you.

So, we mentioned that part of what will help you lose weight is the Law of Attraction. Of course, this isn't just another "law of attraction book." In this book, we will also bring in the power of hypnosis to help you achieve the results that you are seeking. We will be combining the inherent strength of these two things, namely, the Law of Attraction and hypnosis, to help you achieve the weight you desire.

The Law of Attraction has been extremely popular in recent years due to its appearance in the film and book *The Secret*. In case you are not readily familiar with this term and haven't read our previous book *You Can Attract It*, what is the Law of Attraction? The Law of Attraction is a theory that has been with humans since ancient times. In fact, some of the ideology in the Law of Attraction was originally based in Hinduism. The basic idea behind the law of attraction is that "like attracts like." This is particularly true when it comes to your thinking. What you put out into the universe returns to you. If you want positive things to come into your life, you must think positive thoughts and feel positive emotions.

One of the very exciting things about the Law of Attraction is that it means we attract into our life everything we focus on. Of course, this can have either positive or negative implications. Just like we can draw things we want into our lives, we can also draw things we don't want. If we are thinking about not having something we want and are frustrated about the experience, we are drawing scarcity into our experience. When we think about what we love, we draw more of what we love into our lives.

Many people initially seek out the Law of Attraction when they are trying to achieve success in business or making money. So how would Law of Attraction apply to getting rich? The premise in this case would be that in order to get rich, you must think and feel as though you are already rich. This means that if you want to get rich, but are sitting around counting your pennies, you will not achieve your goal.

People rarely get rich sitting in a crummy apartment with no hopes and dreams, no food in the refrigerator feeling miserable and contemplating their failures. Instead, people get rich by putting positive energy out there. This person would need to dream big dreams, buy clothes that made him or her feel rich, hang out where rich people hang and feel the positive emotions associated with wealth.

If you read the last book we co-authored entitled, "You Can Attract It," you can read more about our stories and how we used the Law of Attraction to make positive and remarkable changes in our own lives. We both focused on what we wanted and used strong emotional energy to attract what we wanted into our lives. At this point, due to the Law of Attraction, we are living our dreams.

So if you are reading this book, you are interested in dropping pounds and reaching and maintaining your optimal state of health. The first step to using the Law of Attraction and hypnosis to achieve your weight loss goals is to make the decision that you definitely do want to drop the pounds. We know this sounds like an obvious question on one level. You may be thinking, "Of course I want to lose weight. Why else would I be reading this book?"

Of course, we all know the facts by now. Being obese puts you at risk for a variety of diseases including high blood pressure, heart disease, stroke, gallstones, and diabetes to name just a few. Obesity has even been shown to contribute to an early death! Doctors chalk the soaring levels of obesity up to eating too much, exercising too little and even genetics.

We all know that diet and exercise can help you lose weight. You certainly didn't need to read this book to find out that fact. And we won't deny this fact either; diet and exercise do indeed help you drop pounds. However, there is a missing key that many exercise experts do not mention. Yes, diet and exercise play a large part, but our thoughts and feelings also control whether we will gain or lose weight. If we do not put the Law of Attraction into motion, all the cutting calories and exercising in the world will not give us the results that we are seeking.

However, making the decision that you want to be thinner takes more than just an offhanded desire. You need to truly commit to this decision. You need to become totally clear that weight loss is what you are achieving today. Further, you need to KNOW that soon you will have the new, thinner body that you desire. And once you have made that decision, you need to start feeling as though you have already achieved that goal.

The point is to take the "wanting" and "desiring" out of the picture. When we experience the emotions of needing and wanting, we are drawing more scarcity to ourselves. When we feel unhappy that we are fat, or are frustrated that the pounds aren't coming off faster, we are automatically drawing things we don't want into our life through the Law of Attraction.

Often people think about what they want, but then immediately throw a negative intention into it. For example, when it comes to weight loss, it is really common for people to think to themselves a statement such as one of the following:

"I want to be thinner... but I can't do it. I love food too much."

"I should really go on a diet, but I hate dieting so much."

"I want to lose weight, but I have terrible metabolism."

"To lose weight you need to exercise. I just don't have the time to fit exercising into my schedule."

Do you see the inherent negativity in these statements? Obviously, these statements do not seem like clear, positive statements of intention. Imagine, for a moment, if you had a slender, gorgeous friend who was also in perfect mental and physical shape. Now imagine this friend uttering one of the statements above. How ridiculous would this sound? Of course, you would rarely hear a gorgeous fit and well-balanced person stating these types of negative declarations. A healthy person's thoughts are aligned with the positive feelings around being at a healthy weight.

Lets say you took this person and force-fed them donuts for 30 days and they gained about 15 pounds. Do you know that the fact of the matter is that they could take those 15 pounds right off? On the other hand, if you tried the same experiment with someone who viewed weight loss as difficult, that person would either retain the 15 pounds or lose just enough weight to keep them at the median level at which they began.

Think about if you had a genie in a bottle that literally did everything that you asked her too. Now imagine making these statements to the genie. You wouldn't quite get what you wanted, would you? For example, you would say, "I want to be thinner…" The genie would hear that part of your sentence and begin to make your desires occur. She would start to set that goal into motion for you.

But then, of course, then she would hear the second part of your sentence, "but I can't do it. I love food too much." At that point, the genie would change her course and *stop* assisting you to lose weight. She would turn around and focus on the part of the sentence. This means she would give you more fattening food to love and not help you lose weight. After all, that is what you said you wanted!

Although thinking about a genie in a bottle is a bit clichéd at this point, this example really does serve to explain how people accidentally self-sabotage themselves. Although they think what they are wishing for is clear, they accidentally negate what they want through how they think. They feel strongly that their desires can come true on one level, but then on another level they feel negative and defeated. When setting your intention to lose weight, you want to avoid accidentally putting negative energy into your thoughts and feelings.

So what would be some good solid intention statements for weight loss? Take a look at the following:

"My body is getting thinner and thinner every day."

"All the food I eat nourishes my body and brings me closer to my weight loss goals."

"I eat what I want and don't gain weight."

"Everywhere I go people admire my body and how thin I am."

Do you see how much more positive and clear these statements are? These are desires that the genie can surely run with. Now is the time to start thinking new types of thoughts. This is especially true when it comes to your body and what weight loss goals you are capable of achieving. Now is the time to get rid of thoughts and feelings that no longer serve you. You should only be thinking thoughts that are reflective of the new healthy and fit body that is coming your way.

At this point, you may be skeptical of this information. Can dropping pounds really be easy? We have been taught since day one that weight loss is hard. And, after all, if it were so easy, why would so many people be spending a small fortune on weight loss products and special weight loss meal plans? We have been taught since our childhood that our ability to lose or gain weight is based on what we eat and how much we exercise. We are not saying that these fundamentals are not also true. Weight loss is guided indeed by food consumption and exercise. These are tools that you can use to influence and control your weight.

However, anyone who has tried to diet knows that there is more to losing weight that just diet and exercise. First of all, losing weight and keeping weight off are two separate matters. If you truly want to keep weight off, you must be sure to take additional measures. Also have you ever had the experience of exercising all the time and changing your diet, only to find that you only dropped one or two pounds? No doubt the feeling of stepping on the scale hungry from the days of starvation and achy from all the relentless exercising only to find that you have dropped only half a pound is a frustrating feeling. Many dieters have this experience and end up throwing in the towel.

The reason that the above described scenario happens is that people may be taking the physical actions to lose weight, namely reducing their calories and exercising, yet they have not yet adjusted their mind to the task. Plus, many people who struggle with their weight have had years of negative programming around the issue. As a result, they have negative emotions and fears tied in with losing weight. For many, it's not as easy as snapping your fingers and making these negative associations go away.

Here are some statements that you may have heard early on in your life that may still be lingering in your subconscious:

"Make sure you clean your plate. There are children starving in China."

"You are such a pig!"

"You are not meant to be one of those thin people. You are too big boned."

"You aren't going to lose weight through dieting. You are just meant to be overweight."

Even getting picked last for a team in elementary school can still have ramifications in how we feel about exercising. On a subconscious level, we may feel as though we are not up to the task of losing weight and much of this feeling may be based upon some random incident from our childhood. Once these types of modes of thinking and feeling are set for us, it often is difficult to change and adjust them later.

Here is where hypnosis comes into the picture. Yes, the Law of Attraction will always work to help people lose weight. However, if there are emotional blocks in the way, our results with the Law of Attraction are going to reflect those blocks. Many people struggle to use the Law of Attraction for years with no success. On paper, they are doing everything correctly. They are visualizing their goals, they are feeling the positive emotions, and they are trusting in the universe to deliver their goals. Yet their goals just do not seem to be manifesting as quickly as they should.

In these cases, hypnosis could be what quickly and easily changes this whole picture for them. Steve has had clients that he has worked with that through just one or two hypnosis sessions break through these types of emotional blocks. After that point, it is smooth sailing. Similarly, many people have told Steve that they have had these types of experiences as a result of listening to his hypnosis mp3s.

Stop Telling Yourself You are on a Diet

Its time to make the decision to never tell yourself that you are on a diet again. Sounds pretty good, right? When you say you are dieting, you automatically bring up a wide range of emotions and negative feelings that go along with this word. I am going to go on a diet is in and of itself a very negative goal to be pursuing.

Try saying the word "dieting" out loud. Do you sense how negative this word can be? When you tell someone that you are dieting, they will also automatically conjure up negative thoughts in their own minds as well. Also people tend to assume dieting is hard. It is maybe even impossible. We want you to let go of that feeling and instead start believing that achieving your new weight is easy.

When you tell yourself that you are on a diet, you can automatically dredge up a variety of painful and frustrating feelings. The word also implies that you will be denying yourself things that you like. The more that you equate your journey with the negative connotations of the word "diet", the harder it will be to reach your goals. After all, like attracts like, so the more you focus on this negative term, the more negative experiences will accompany your experience.

When you use the word diet, you instantly start thinking about the things you will be denied. All of a sudden, you are struck with the impossibility of the situation. After all, food will certainly be presented before you in the coming weeks, and you so you will start thinking about how you will have to deny yourself everything. This can be a very painful feeling.

In fact, starting the very next day when you go to work perhaps there will be something like donuts or candy at your office. Some offices, in fact, keep big jars of candy on hand. When you walk by someone's desk, certainly they will try to offer you some candy or, worse yet, a donut. Or it will be someone's birthday perhaps, and you will be offered a big piece of cake. Immediately, the horror of the situation may set in. You may think, "I am on a diet. I will have to deny myself these pleasures."

Immediately a host of negative feelings may be triggered as a result. All of these feelings can bring a lot of negative experiences due to the Law of Attraction. For example, you might start thinking, "I can never do it." " This is too hard." "Is dieting really worth depriving myself of these pleasures." All of these thoughts and feelings will bring you more deprivation and less success via the Law of Attraction.

Similarly, telling yourself and others that you are going to "lose weight" is also not the best word choice. The reason for this is that everyone knows on a subconscious level that if you lose something you must try and find it.

Many Law of Attraction experts speculate that when it comes to weight loss this is the reason why so many people gain the weight back again.

In order to make the Law of Attraction work on your behalf, just go ahead and pick a different phrase. Try to make the phrase something that gets you excited and feeling motivated. If your phrase conjures up positive images of your new slimmer body that is even better.

Here are some examples that you can choose from:

- *I am getting healthier*
- *I am burning fat*
- *I am reaching my ideal weight*
- *I am getting in touch with a new, slimmer me*
- *I am reaching radiant health*

Or go ahead and choose your own positive, affirming statement. Trust us, if you are serious about dropping pounds, taking the words "diet" and "losing weight" out of your vocabulary will do you a great service.

... taking the words "diet" and "losing weight" out of your vocabulary will do you a great service.

There is another factor at hand as well. Many people who crave desserts and fattening foods are also addicted to these foods. Studies prove that you can get addicted to sugar. For example, according to researches at The University of Bordeaux in France, sugar is more addictive than cocaine! Rats were allowed to choose between water sweetened with sugar versus water sweetened with cocaine. The majority of rats preferred the water with the sugar.

You can also certainly get addicted to chemicals and preservatives in a host of junk food. Part of the problem with the initial stages of your "diet" is that not only are you depriving yourself of foods you love; you are also breaking an addiction and going through some withdrawal symptoms.

So instead of focusing on the foods you will be denied at work, change your thinking to the more positive goal. For example, if your goal for the week is not "I will stick to my diet" but instead "I will achieve radiant health," you will be far more likely to make the best decisions. You will also be more likely to experience positive, hopeful feelings in the process.

Instead of thinking, "how will I resist the donuts?" instead change your thinking to something like "I can't wait until lunch when I can crunch on the beautiful red peppers I brought from the farmer's market!" Think to yourself a positive affirmation such as "the piece of organic chocolate that I savor at the end of the day is really going to be divine and will fill my body full of antioxidants." The trick is to gradually begin seeing food in a whole new way. Once you have changed your approach to being healthy, the pounds will drop right off.

This book will show you how to harness the Law of Attraction and use it to your benefit to lose weight. We will take you through the entire process of what you need to do, eat and think. In the final chapter of the book, we also present some of our favorite recipes that will keep you excited to cook and eat healthy meals. Whether you are looking to eat right, get motivated or just see weight loss results, this book will help you achieve these goals.

Chapter 2

COMPONENTS OF A HYPNOSIS SESSION

"Every day in every way, I am getting better and better." —Emile Coue

Before we get too far into our exploration of the Law of Attraction and how it can help you lose weight, lets take a moment and explore hypnotism. Hypnotism is also an effective way in allowing you to make a positive change and get rid of habits and behaviors that are holding you back from your ultimate success. Because hypnotism is so powerful in helping people achieve weight loss results, it only makes sense to include some information in this book about how it can help you.

We are huge believers in the fact that sometimes hypnosis is the quickest and easiest way to get you to achieve your goals. In fact, you can always hire a hypnotist like Steve to guide you through the process. Incidentally, one of the issues that his clients book him for most is for those looking to lose weight. Other reasons that people see a hypnotist like Steve would be for issues like smoking, anxiety, phobias, anger management, and nail biting, to name just a few conditions. Steve has found through the years that when he uses hypnotherapy to treat these sorts of issues as well as others, the results are nothing short of amazing.

If you are reading this book, you likely also realize that hypnotherapy is a very serious and effective way to help people achieve their goals and clear blocks. It is nothing at all similar to the stage hypnosis you may have seen where people are forced to make fools out of themselves acting like a chicken and kissing complete strangers. In hypnotherapy all the suggestions that are made to your unconscious mind are positive, and they are all designed to help you.

One of the great things about hypnosis is that this process guides you to being able to control your thoughts and feelings. This sort of discipline over one's thoughts works hand in hand with the Law of Attraction. As we know, our thoughts create our reality. So why not guide them in the best direction possible with the assistance of hypnosis? In fact, hypnosis is one of the most effective tools that you can use in jump-starting the Law of Attraction to take you where you want to go in your life. And hypnosis and hypnotherapy is available for you anytime. In fact, you can even hypnotize yourself and you don't even need to leave the comfort of your own home or meet personally with a hypnotist.

There are ample methods by which you can hypnotize yourself. This process is called "self hypnosis." Self-hypnosis can also produce quick results. You can, of course, find a wide variety of self-hypnosis products at Steve's website http://www.stevegjones.com. Audio mp3s and CDs are an easy and cost effective way of hypnotizing yourself. The topics of these audio self-hypnosis products widely range and include everything from avoiding panic attacks and helping insomnia to curing depression and stopping jealousy.

Lets take a moment and explore how the process of how hypnosis works.

Induction

What is induction? A hypnotic induction is the suggestions that occur at the beginning of your session. In other words, an induction "induces" you to become hypnotized. When you first think of the word induction, what might first come to man is an image of a man with a swinging pendulum saying, "You are getting very sleepy." Often a bright object held 10 inches or so away from the eyes is in fact one way to perform an induction. The client fixes his eyes upon that one object. As a result, the pupils dilate and the eyelids end up closing.

This technique of hypnotic induction is commonly seen in movies and TV. James Braid developed this method of hypnotizing someone. In fact, many people call this method, which deals with fixating the eyes, "Braidism." However, in reality, few hypnotists actually swing a pendulum before your eyes.

Hippolyte Bernheim later popularized the method of focusing on a verbal suggestion instead of just something physical like a pendulum. Bernheim published the book "Suggesting Therapeutics: A Treatise on the Nature and Use of Hypnotism." This book emphasized how powerful mental suggestion can be for hypnotizing people.

Actually there are a host of different techniques for induction that are used by hypnotists. Some popular methods include the following:

- **The Arm Drop Method**

  The client is asked to raise his right hand above his head. At this moment, he is given a suggestion. The downward movement of the arm is tied into going into a relaxed state.

- **The Direct Gaze Induction**

  The hypnotist stares at the client directly in his or her eye during the induction.

- **The Hand Shake Method**

  The client is seated in a chair. The hypnotist reaches out his or her hand and gets the client to shake hands and slowly begins moving the hand up and down.

- **The Fixation Object Method**

  This is the traditional method of induction we discussed above. The client is asked to stare fixedly at an object without losing focus. A shiny object is used.

- **Relaxation Induction**

  The client is taken through a series of verbal suggestions that allow him or her to become progressively more and more relaxed.

- **The Confusion Method**

  In this method of hypnotic induction, the hypnotist intentionally confuses the client. This confusion causes the brain to go looking internally for answers and causes the person to go into a trance. Milton Erickson is initially credited with this method. One way to use the confusion method is through what is called pattern interruption. This would be done through setting up a client's expectations for what he or she would normally do and say, and then doing otherwise.

When it comes to self-hypnosis, obviously you don't have a hypnotist physically in front of you to guide you through the process. The induction usually tends to be a series of verbal suggestions and deep breathing exercises that allow you to become progressively more and more relaxed. It is also important to be in a position that is very comfortable and relaxing for you at the start of the session.

The book *Clinical and Experimental Hypnosis in Medicine, Dentistry, and Psychology* by William S. Kroger and Michael D Yapko describes the best method for the hypnotist to handle the induction period. "Before beginning an induction procedure, the operator should describe as simply as possible what he is going to do, what the subject is supposed to feel, and what is expected of him-this raises the expectancy level. The operator must stress that the more attention the subject directs to his suggestions, the more successful the induction will be."

Another important thing to note about induction is that the hypnotist must be extremely confident in his or her abilities. If the client senses any weakness or uncertainty in the thoughts or behavior of the hypnotist, the induction is less likely to work. Therefore, if you go to see a good hypnotist or hypnotherapist, you should expect that he or she would act very confident and secure.

Deepening

Deepening is the part of hypnosis that causes a person to go into a deeper state of relaxation towards the hypnotic state. The most common method of deepening is for the hypnotist to suggest counting down your state of relaxation. With each number, you can go deeper into relaxation. This technique also works quite well for self-hypnosis. With each breath you can go deeper and deeper into the hypnotic state. Another method of deepening is imagining yourself going down a staircase. These are just two deepening techniques, but they are two of the most popular.

What is interesting is that it is never the hypnotist who truly guides the client into hypnosis. The person being hypnotized actually guides his or her own mind towards this state. Becoming naturally relaxed is what enables the mind to eventually slip into a trance. This is one of the reasons that self-hypnosis works so well. You don't actually need a hypnotist present to become hypnotized. Your mind can do the work on its own.

Deepening is somewhat like falling asleep in that you can't force yourself to experience it. You could stay up for hours trying to force yourself to fall asleep. The mind often won't allow it if you are trying too hard. Instead, the deepening is something that occurs naturally. You will not be able to physically control whether or not it happens. Instead, it is just something that results from a suggestion.

Guided imagery can work extremely well for deepening. As we mentioned above, walking down a staircase works very well. Other good ideas for guided imagery include going down an escalator or an elevator. Some types of deepening imagery work best with certain types of people. If you are doing self-hypnosis, you may need to experiment to find the type of deepening exercises that work best for you.

Script

A hypnotic script is the text that guides the client through the hypnosis session. This is perhaps the most important element of hypnosis. Hypnotic scripts can vary quite widely. They can be quite simple or very complex. Sometimes hypnotic scripts even embed commands or embed guided visualization.

The point is that the script delivers an important message to your subconscious mind. This is the message that will begin to change the way that you think and feel for the better. The script is the core of the hypnosis experience.

When you see a hypnotist, he or she doesn't just read these words off a sheet of paper. The script is spoken directly to the client. In fact, this script may change depending on the reaction he or she is getting during the session. In this way, the process is somewhat improvisational. Even though the client is in a trance, the hypnotist will still be getting non-verbal cues as to how to proceed with the script. In other words, good hypnotists will not simply be reading the same text he or she reads for every other client. The session will be specifically targeted to your needs.

A script's text will often include NLP or Neuro Linguistic Programming. NLP uses language techniques and patterns to guide you towards the desired result. The end result of the script is that new patterns are formed in your mind.

If you decide to get an mp3 for self-hypnosis to lose weight, the script will suggest positive changes in your life that will take you towards that goal. The mp3 will influence your mind in a deep unconscious level. The actual experience will seem to you very much like daydreaming. Some people compare getting hypnotized to getting lost in a movie or television program. You will focus intensely on the information you are receiving and you will tune out everything else.

Everything in a good hypnosis script will impact your subconscious in a positive manner. If you want to check out some actual scripts for yourself, you can find books of some of the best hypnotic scripts at www.stevegjones.com.

With some experience, you can eventually start writing your own scripts to be used during self-hypnosis. There are many ways you can use hypnosis for your success. It is a journey; so don't feel as though you have to initially understand everything about it. Just start taking small steps towards making steps towards using hypnosis to make a positive change for yourself.

Amnesia

Hypnotic amnesia is when a hypnotist or hypnotherapist suggests that the end of the session the client should forget some of the work that is done. This is important because it will keep the rational mind from analyzing too intensely what has happened. The goal is to let the subconscious mind rest with the work that has been done. If the rational mind interferes with scrutiny, it can interfere with the results. This is especially true for people who tend to be highly analytical.

Now if a hypnotist or hypnotherapist induces amnesia, does that mean you are going to start forgetting everything in your life including your past memories? Luckily, the answer to this question is not at all. If that were the case, hypnosis would clearly be much less popular. Hypnotic amnesia is only very temporary. In fact, later on you will be able to recall more of what occurred in your session. Again, the point of post-hypnotic suggestion is to keep the client's mind from immediately analyzing and deconstructing what just happened.

Trance Termination

Trance termination is bringing someone out of the trance safely. Often you see this done in the movies or television with the simple snap of the hypnotist's fingers. In hypnotherapy, the trance termination process is often more detailed.

The hypnotherapist will make suggestions to review what has gone on in the session and to reiterating how these skills can be used in the client's daily life. The hypnotherapist also mentions that this information is now readily accessible to the client whenever he or she needs it. At this point, the client's awareness is gradually brought back to the present.

The process of trance termination is important because it guides a person back into day-to-day consciousness. A hypnotherapist certainly wouldn't want to send a person out the door and into their car to drive home while they were still in the hypnotic state! This could lead to a potentially dangerous car ride home.

The unconscious mind also needs time to firmly implant the new ideas and suggestions. If you use a recording for self-hypnosis, the voice on the recording will gradually bring you out of the hypnotic state. It will remind you that your mind is awake and alert.

Self-Hypnosis

So what are the advantages of going to a hypnotist or hypnotherapist as opposed to trying self-hypnosis? In reality, both processes have their own advantages. When you see a hypnotherapist, the session will be more oriented towards you personally. On the other hand, a self-hypnosis mp3 will be more general. When the session is more geared towards your individual issues and concerns, the session can be more powerful and focused.

For example, if you cannot stop eating doughnuts at work when your coworker brings them to the office, you can tell your hypnotist that information ahead of time. As a result, he or she can incorporate that information into your hypnosis script and guide you through the process of making better choices rather than eating doughnuts.

On the other hand, a self-hypnosis mp3 will make suggestions that are more general and would apply for a wide array of people.

Also often people find that they lack the discipline to effectively perform self-hypnosis on themselves. When you are trying to make positive changes at home, it is easy to forget or procrastinate. Even if you have bought a self-hypnosis mp3, your unconscious mind might resist letting you listen to it regularly.

On the other hand, if you make an appointment with a hypnotist or hypnotherapist for a phone session or office visit, there is a good chance that you will go and keep your appointment. In this way, seeing a hypnotist or hypnotherapist in person has a definite edge.

There are times, however, where learning self-hypnosis would come in extremely handy. For example, women are having great results with learning this technique to help during pregnancy and childbirth. Learning self-hypnosis can be especially necessary during natural childbirth where the mother isn't given painkillers that a hospital might offer.

Psychology Today recently wrote about the power of self-hypnosis to assist during childbirth in an article called "Labor Pain Made Easy with Self-Hypnosis." Author Steven Gurgevich writes, "'Pain' is the word most associated with labor and delivery. But it doesn't have to be; here's why. Learning self-hypnosis can make childbirth and labor much easier with less discomfort, more control and self-confidence. Here is a list of just some of the many benefits of learning self-hypnosis during pregnancy."

Knowing self-hypnosis techniques can provide women with a variety of advantages. They can more effectively relax and reduce their stress around childbirth. They can also learn to control their body through self-hypnosis with control over the cervix, control over experiencing sensory reactions, and enhancing their ability to detach from the pain.

Obviously, if self-hypnosis can work for childbirth, it can also help for a wide range of issues. This includes, of course, becoming healthier. Various experts have addressed the beneficial nature of self-hypnosis for weight loss.

For example, in a 2004 issue of *Oprah Magazine* the article mentioned, "clients who learned self-hypnosis lost twice as much weight as those who didn't." The National Women's Health Resource Center stated, "As a relaxation technique, hypnosis can help reduce your stress. It's also used to relieve phobias, lessen anxiety, break addictions and to ease symptoms of conditions such as asthma or allergy. Using hypnosis can help patients control nausea and vomiting from cancer medications and morning sickness, reduce bleeding during surgery, steady the heartbeat and bring down blood pressure."

Another great thing about understanding self-hypnosis or having mp3s and audios readily available is that it is a great way to snap yourself out of a negative mental state. It is a quick fix that is quite effective and works pretty much immediately.

When you are working to produce good results in your life with the Law of Attraction, it is a great idea to have a tool like hypnosis that can keep you on track. We can't feel 100% perfect all of the time. At some point, situations are inevitably going to arise that upset us. However, if we have tools in our pocket that can guide us to a positive mental state, it can be extremely empowering. These

... if we have tools in our pocket that can guide us to a positive mental state, it can be extremely empowering.

tools will also assure that you don't get off-track in your quest to get healthy. And the healthier you become, the easier it will be to stay positive and motivated.

Before you begin any kind of hypnosis, whether traditional hypnosis, hypnotherapy or self-hypnosis, it is important to determine exactly what you want to get out of the process. This comes back to the importance of establishing your goals and desires for your end result. This is important to establish not only to allow the Law of Attraction to work on your behalf, but also to make sure you achieve your goals through hypnosis or self-hypnosis sessions.

When it comes to hypnosis, the simpler your goal the better. Even if you have tons of issues you want to work on eventually, it is best to focus on one goal at a time. This way your unconscious mind will not get confused.

For example, you could start with losing weight or getting healthier. Once you feel as though that goal has been achieved or is well underway, next you could move on to something like quitting smoking. Once you have effectively quit smoking, then you could work on your fear of flying and so on.

Chapter 3

THE SIX STEPS OF YOU CAN ATTRACT IT

"Your imagination is your preview of life's coming attractions." —*Albert Einstein*

In our last book You Can Attract It, we discussed six steps that are important to take towards attracting the life of your dreams. In this book, we wanted to elaborate on these six steps. We also wanted to discuss how specifically these steps can be applied towards your new desired weight. If you have already read *You Can Attract It*, don't skip this chapter because this book contributes a lot more to the topic and this will be essential to begin your process.

Step One: Changing Your Negative Powers into Positive Powers

You have four powers that are important to always remember when you are using the Law of Attraction for losing weight. These powers are your thoughts, emotions, visualizations and your actions. Even though the word "powers" may sound a bit extreme, you really do have these powers at your disposal and like the powers of any good superhero, they can change reality. We choose the term powers to stress just how magnificent and transformative these abilities are!

Here is how the path you need to take to allow these four emotions to lead directly to permanent weight loss:

1. **Cultivate new thoughts around the topic of losing weight.**

   In other words, if you have been thinking all of your life that losing weight is impossible, let go of that habit. Change your thoughts into new production ones that will support your weight loss goals.

2. **Feel new positive emotions around the issue of fat**

   Do you have strong, negative emotions that are tied up with the theme of weight loss? Some people say that they look at their own bodies in the mirror with disgust and anger. Others say they hate themselves for not having a beautiful slim body. When you are using the four powers to lose weight, you will need to release all of your negative emotions around losing weight. Make sure that you feed yourself with positive, fulfilling emotions about your body and your success. These negative emotions will only draw you further away from the new body you desire.

3. **Visualize your powerful, strong, thin new body**

   Stop looking in the mirror and think negative thoughts about your body. Once you have ceased cultivating a negative self-image, you can finally start allowing new visualizations about your appearance and health come through.

   Here are a few more examples: Have you ever gone shopping, seen some clothing you really love, but then said to yourself, "I will never fit into that. I am too fat." If you have, you need to change those sorts of counterproductive visions of yourself. Instead of negating your ability to lose weight, that situation would actually be the perfect time to use positive visualizations to your benefit. Instead, go ahead and visualize yourself wearing that outfit and feel the feelings of how good you will look. Think about yourself walking down the street wearing those clothes and how good you will look. Try to bring as many details into this visualization as possible.

4. **Start practicing new positive actions around your weight loss goals**

   The next power at your disposal is that of action. This means that in addition to thinking, feeling and visualizing positively about weight loss, you must also begin to take the steps to have a new healthy thin body. You are probably expecting for this to be the part of the book where we insist that you go on a starvation diet and wake up early to exercise for an hour at the gym every morning before work. The fact of the matter is that *this isn't* what we are suggesting. Well… we aren't, of course, unless you want to go that down that route. In that case, by all means go work out all day long at the gym. But it really isn't necessary. Remember, we are focusing on keeping everything easy.

Your positive actions need to come from you. They also need to feel fulfilling and inspiration for you to practice. So, in other words, killing yourself at the gym isn't really going to help you lose weight in the long run unless you feel good about it. Some people, in fact, enjoy that sort of exercise routine. Everyone is different, so you need to take some time and explore what specific types of actions you enjoy.

The key here is to start practicing actions around losing weight that feel good to you. Now this also doesn't mean that you should go out and buy a big jelly doughnut every night and eat it. After all, that would not feel good to you in the long run. Although you may enjoy this routine at first, eating jelly doughnuts every night is not a sustainable habit that is going to help you feel good for long. Sugar causes immediate energy rushes and then sharp negative crashes afterwards. Sugar also depletes our immune system and makes us susceptible to illness. The list of ailments caused by sugar goes on and on.

First, it is necessary to achieve a state of balance and awareness when it comes to your body. Once you reach that state, you will no longer truly want to cultivate habits that don't support your health and fitness goals. At this point, once all of your 4 powers are truly in alignment, you will no longer crave unhealthy habits. You will see these cravings disappear little by little until they are gone for good.

Step 2: Know What You Do Not Want

Before you get to the point where you focus on what you do want, it is important to take some time and really examine what you do not want. It is time to really dig deep and focus on yourself. We are sometimes so overwhelmed with messages from the media and from others in our lives, we don't take time to stop and ask ourselves what we really want.

Now ask yourself the question, "Do I really want to lose weight?" Now at first your automatic response to this question may be, "Of course I want to lose weight! Why else would I have purchased this book?" However, the fact of the matter is that it is possible you are honing in on what other people want, and not your own true desires. There are actually many people out there who are obese that are satisfied with their weight. If you are one of those people, you can follow all the weight loss plans in the world, but you will most likely not successfully drop pounds. In this case, you want to be at your current obese weight, so you will stay there.

Here is another less dramatic example. Often women feel forced to lose weight to please their husbands or boyfriends. Lets take a woman named Peggy. Peggy is happy and content with her body. She is about 10 pounds overweight and a bit chubby around her midsection. But truly, these extra ten pounds do not bother her. Now her husband Bill has been badgering her for years to get back to the perfect weight she was at when they first got married 20 years ago. After hearing Bill pressure her relentlessly, she finally gives in and tells him she will drop the 10 pounds. She tells him she will fit back into her wedding dress in the next month. She promises to go on a strict diet.

If you are like Peggy and losing weight to please someone else and not yourself, it is going to be much harder to achieve this goal. In order to line up your 4 powers of manifestation, your desires have to be truly aligned with your body, mind and spirit.

Make sure that what you are intending to achieve is what you truly want. As for Peggy, perhaps what she really wants is not necessarily to lose the ten pounds, but instead to just get stronger and feel more flexible. Every time she drives by the yoga studio, she thinks to herself, "I would love to learn yoga." She often fantasizes about training to run a marathon in her city, but never does it. So Peggy actually does have health and fitness aspirations that really get her motor running. It is just that Peggy really doesn't care what the scale says like her husband does. In this particular scenario, what should Peggy do? Of course, she should follow her own hopes and desires and ignore her husband's fixation on the scale. Now perhaps when she gets more fit and strong, the weight loss will follow as a side benefit. But truly, Peggy needs to focus on what gets her excited and invigorated.

Not everyone is going to have the same weight loss goals. And the same specifics aren't going to work for every person. That is why we would never tell you to go on a specific diet plan or particular fitness plan. While one person might lose 30 pounds through following some famous diet book and never gain the weight back, another person may attempt the same diet and gain 30 pounds.

Be sure to eliminate from your diet plan anything that you do not truly want. Otherwise you will get steered in the wrong direction. Do not follow a certain diet because someone else says you should or because you feel outside pressure to do so. The diet that is going to give you results is the one that is best aligned with your own personal imprint and level of motivation. And if you decide that you are completely happy with your current weight and do not want to change, feel free to put this book down now.

Step 3: Know What You Do Want

Ok, so you are still reading... You have decided you definitely do want to achieve a new healthier weight. It is now time to get as clear as possible. Now is the time to shift away from what you do not want and start focusing on your own unique vision.

Yes, we did define that you want to drop pounds. But that statement is very general. Lets get more specifically focused in on what you really want.

According to the Law of Attraction, the images in your mind are the ones that you will be drawing to you. Imagine exactly what weight you want to be. In fact, come up with a specific amount of pounds you want to weigh. Know exactly what size pants you want to be wearing. Take a moment and see a specific image of what you will look like in a bathing suit. If its fitness you are looking to achieve, imagine the physical feats you will be capable of. Will you be able to swim across a lake? Hike a 6-mile trail in an afternoon? What will that feel like? The more detail that you can add into the vision of what you want, the better.

Now ask yourself why you want to lose weight. Get in touch with all the positive emotions associated with what you want. How wonderful will it feel wearing that bathing suit on the beach? What will it feel like to have that firm healthy body? If you want to lose weight to attract a significant other into your life, go ahead and let yourself feel the emotions of how wonderful and fulfilling this relationship will be. Imagine the warm embrace of holding this person in your arms and watching as he or she admires your new thin, fit body. It is important to get in touch with these emotions and how they will transform your life.

Step 4: Ask for It

Now that you have gotten clear on what you do not want, and what you do not, it is time to simply ask for what you want. Yes, its true that it is this simple. Yes, asking for what we want seems like the easiest thing to do in the world. We knew how to ask for things when were just babies. We asked for the milk or we asked for the pacifier, and it magically appeared. However, somewhere between the time we were babies and the present moment, we forgot how to ask for things. This is usually due to some disappointments that occurred in our lives that made us give up on our own natural abilities to manifest what we want and need. Often people have such a difficult time asking for what they want. In fact, Steve frequently offers hypnosis to help people achieve just that goal.

But most people do have the natural capability to just simply ask for what they want. Just be careful to not fall into the trap of thinking or feeling negative emotion when you ask. Make sure your requests are straightforward and positive. Don't ask for something and then negative it afterwards by thinking, "this is impossible," or "this will never work." Simple ask the universe to bring you what you want, and then leave it at that.

Now once you have gotten used to asking the universe to deliver you your weight loss goals, go ahead and ask every day. When you ask, make sure deep down you will actually receive these goals. Now we all have heard the stories of people who have tried to lose weight and failed. When you are asking for what you want, do not allow these stories to enter into your mind. Make sure you remain positive and never get frustrated. Even if you have asked to lose weight for the 30th day in a row and not dropped one pound, be sure to remain free of agitation or frustration. You must keep your faith that the Law of Attraction is delivering what you have asked for.

Step 5: Allow It

The fifth step in the law of attraction process is to allow your new slimmer body and fitness goals to come to you. Just telling yourself that you are allowing and ready to lose the weight isn't enough. You need to truly embrace this new reality with your entire being. You need to trust 100% and be committed to the fact that soon the new weight that you desire will indeed be yours.

Many people suffer from self-esteem issues and these negative thoughts can block them from properly allowing their success. Make sure that you understand that you deserve to lose weight and be thin. You deserve to be at the most optimal state of health possible. You are already beautiful. You are physically fit. And you are successful. You already possess these traits, now is the time to manifest them into reality. All you need to do is open your door and allow the success to unfold in your life.

Remember to consistently focus on what you do want. Keep your mind away from what you do not want at all times. Anytime that you begin to feel frustrated or anxious, just be sure to relax and focus wholeheartedly on what you desire. It is much easier to lose weight when you accept and love yourself. This is yet another reason why negative chatter to yourself is counterproductive.

Also the more anxiety you feel, the more likely you may be to eat foods that are not nourishing for your body. That is why often people gorge themselves on junk food when they feel miserable and anxious. They aren't just eating the food because they like the taste or because they feel hungry. People often use unhealthy foods almost as a drug. Often they feel lonely, unattractive or unworthy, and they try to feel the void with food. But at the same time, they are feeding the negativity. This is the Law of Attraction in action. When people feel at their lowest, they often eat the unhealthiest food that will potentially harm their body. This is the process like attracts like that we keep referring to.

Consider the following scenario: Sandy has a miserable stressful day; perhaps she loses her job and has a fight with her boyfriend. Her emotions spiral downward quickly and she feels as though she is on the brink of an emotional breakdown. She comes home feeling terrible about herself and her life, she opens the refrigerator and pulls out… a big plate of salad. Of course, this story sounds silly. In actuality, Sandy would probably be getting a big plate of pasta, ice cream or pie.

Can you see how the negative feelings always tend to manifest themselves in destructive eating habits? By eating the ice cream or pizza and not supporting healthy feelings and habits, Sandy is sabotaging her success on her diet. But this event is a direct result of her negative feelings and stress.

Always Feel Grateful

Another important part to the process is to always be grateful. Think about your life in general and what you appreciate. Consider your family, your friendships, your job, your health, and other areas of life that you appreciate. When you think about these elements of your life that are going well, really feel how happy they make you. As humans, we all tend to take certain parts of our lives for granted. This just happens so don't blame yourself. Try for a minute to look at your life with fresh eyes and consider all of the wonderful things you get to experience every day. Is the sun shining? Is it beautiful outside? Do you happen to have a cute and faithful pet dog or cat to keep you company? All of these are examples of things you have which can fill your life with joy.

Many people who are overweight and struggling get so caught up in the issue of their weight. They begin to lose touch with the big picture and all that there is to be happy about, whether they are the perfect weight or obese. Even if you are currently 50, 60, 70 pounds overweight or more, there is still plenty to be grateful about.

Even those who are at a very unhealthy weight have plenty about which they can be grateful. Are you able to go out and exercise? More than likely, you can do some form of exercise. And does your body know how to burn and process fat? Most likely it does do so automatically. Do you enjoy healthy nutritious food? Certainly there is some healthy food that you love eating. Do you enjoy drinking a big cold glass of water? Yes? Great! Water is excellent for your body and drinking lots of water each day supports your fat burning goals. Instead of feeling negative about your current weight situation, try to focus in on how lucky you are to have so many things that are going right in your life.

You can look at every negative situation when it comes to your weight and body and turn it around into something you are grateful for. Being grateful is so important because it puts you in a positive reception state that will allow better things to come into your life.

The Power of Hypnosis and Affirmations

Hypnosis is extremely helpful for raising self-esteem. If you feel as though you are experiencing too much negativity, try hypnosis mp3s. Self-hypnosis is always at your disposal and it is free to use. It is not as though you have to hire a professional hypnotist every time you want to positively readjust your subconscious mind. Gaining control over your subconscious can be achieved. At this point, the Law of Attraction can work in a faster and more fluid manner.

Even reading a positive affirmation script in front of a mirror can be enormously helpful. Tell yourself that you are powerful, beautiful and thin. Recognize that day-by-day you are getting thinner and healthier. Breathe in and out and try to release the stressful chatter in your mind. Breathe deeply, Repeat to yourself that you are a strong, beautiful and successful person who can achieve whatever you dream of.

When you are telling yourself positive affirmations, also acknowledge that the Law of Attraction is working perfectly in your life. At this point, you have already accomplished the first few steps of the six steps of *You Can Attract It*. You have changed your negative powers into new positive ones. You have gotten clear on what you want, and what you do not want. And then you have asked for what you want. The process of allowing should in fact be the most enjoyable.

However, often people find it difficult to relax because they feel as though they need to do something. And they find it hard to trust that everything is exactly as it should be. Make sure that you remember that everything is perfect. Again, reading a script to yourself can be extremely helpful in getting to the perfect state of allowing.

It is important to recognize that you have the ability to allow amazing things into your life. Remember that you do not have to do anything to allow. Now is your opportunity to be at peace. You can just relax and let your new thin body arrive.

Create room in your life for the new positive energy and the healthy new you. How do you create this room? You do it by feeling wholeheartedly as though you deserve to lose weight.

Often dieters start out motivated and doing great using the Law of Attraction to lose weight, but then give up during the stage of allowing. After all, they have done the work deciding what they want, visualizing and using their positive powers, shouldn't the pounds just be dropping off effortlessly? Sometimes yes. Sometimes the pounds take a bit longer to drop. The important thing is to not give up. It is crucial at this stage to keep thinking positive thoughts and resisting any urges to get negative.

Step 6: Receive It, Enjoy It, Be Thankful for It, Surround Yourself with It

The final step of the process is fairly self-explanatory. Once you have achieved your new desired weight, Receive It, Enjoy It, Be Thankful for It, and Surround Yourself with It. Feeling these positive emotions are key. You have done it! You have decided on a goal, set it into motion and they reaped the positive results. This is no small matter and you should give yourself a pat on the back! Even if it took far longer than you expected to lose weight, this does not minimize the results. You did lose the weight all the same and that was your goal!

Part of the reason it is so important to celebrate and rejoice at this stage of the game is that you need to continue to appreciate the Law of Attraction and how well it works. Also now is not the time to revert back to old negative patterns. Through your weight loss journey, you were able to set up new powerful milestones in your life. And you have been able to embrace your health and vitality in the process.

So you are now at the weight you have been hoping for. Now its time to start enjoying! Make sure you buy some of the clothes you dreamed about wearing. Why not take a trip to the beach and feel how wonderful it is to wear a swimsuit you previously would not have imagined? Feel free to enjoy your new appearance and the admiring gazes from other people. You did the work and you deserve this.

When you eat healthy food that is nutrition and revitalizing to your body, feel how good you feel eating this food. Make sure you take time to thank yourself for treating your body so well. When you pass up food that is fattening and detrimental for your health, give yourself kudos for making such a smart life-affirming decision. You are contributing to your health and well-being and that is something to celebrate.

Whatever exercise you have chosen to do to contribute to your weight loss goals, make sure that you enjoy it. Appreciate how much easier physical fitness is for you now than when you weighed more. Do you feel lighter and freer when you exercise? Can you run or swim faster? Perhaps you even have more energy in general to achieve good in other parts of your life?

All of these are successes that are to be appreciated and never overlooked. After all, these achievements were the direct result of your positive thinking, positive actions. The Law of Attraction is doing its job to make your life better. Cherish how wonderful it is to be in excellent health.

In being thankful for these achievements, make sure you thank the universe everyday for what you have achieved. Even if you have only lost 5 pounds and have 35 more to lose, thank the universe for the weight that you have lost thus far. Remind yourself that you are losing weight faster and more productively all the time. When you look at yourself in the mirror, feel free to utter out loud "Thank you." You can also just think these words silently to yourself. Every time you think "Thank You," you send positive vibrations out to the universe. These feelings tell the universe you are grateful, acknowledge the Law of Attraction and are ready to receive new amazing things in your life.

By the phrase "Surround Yourself with It," we mean that you should be sure to nourish your health and weight loss by spending times in environments that are supportive of these goals. In other words, once you have lost the weight, you probably don't want to spend your afternoons hanging out in a dive bar or a greasy diner.

As much as you can, make your outdoor environments match your feelings and emotions inside. If you have friends that enjoy pigging out every weekend, you may have to start distancing yourself from these friends. Instead try to find a new healthy environment that is more in line with your new thoughts and beliefs. Perhaps you can find a healthy restaurant, a beautiful park or a yoga studio to spend more of your time.

The six steps outlined in this chapter are all very important for your process and success. This is not just your current success, but also your success in the future. If you follow the steps with a great deal of clarity, you will achieve the weight loss results that you are looking for. If for some reason, you have not lost weight as you intended, sit down with yourself and ask yourself if you truly have been avoiding negativity.

Have you been focusing on what you do not want? Even for us, the authors, it took awhile to perfect these six steps to the point where they gave us results every time. We cannot stress enough how important it is to get very clear on what you want. Remember this is not what others have told you that you want, or what you think you want due to peer pressure. You must zero in on what you truly desire. Once you pinpoint this desire, keep this image in your mind at all times.

> We cannot stress enough how important it is to get very clear on what you want.

Chapter 4
CONFIDENCE

"You are the only person on earth who can use your ability." —Zig Ziglar

So much of our success in life is based on confidence. If you constantly doubt yourself or are fearful, it can lead to results you do not want. You are constantly like a magnet, drawing to yourself events and situations that mirror what is going on in the inside. Therefore, people who are insecure tend to attract results that they do not want. When you eat something, you need to be confident that it will be good for your body. When you exercise, be confident that it is just what your body needs.

What is confidence? Confidence doesn't necessarily mean egotistical or condescending behavior. Sometimes when people hear the word "confident," they often perceive it as having a negative meaning. However, the word that should have a negative connotation is arrogant. Sometimes people fail to realize, that in fact, arrogance and self-confidence are quite different. Arrogance actually originates from fear and insecurity. On the other hand, confidence is an inner knowing that you know who you are and where you are going.

Confidence also means that you take responsibility for yourself, and know how to make things happen. People who are truly confident have their goals and dreams in mind and work to make them reality. When you have harnessed the power of the Law of Attraction to work on your behalf, there is no reason not to feel confident and powerful. Of course, hypnosis can take your level of confidence even another step further.

Here is an effective exercise to take a moment out and try. Think about the leaders in the world that you know and admire. Take out a sheet of paper and write down 3 or 4 people that fit into this category. Skip a space between each person's name. These leaders should have traits of confidence that you have seen and that you respect. Now next to each person's name on your paper, write down a few reasons why you think this person is so confident. What does this person do that makes you believe that he or she is confident?

Now reflect on this list for a moment. Could you apply any of these reasons to your own life? If so, circle all the traits that also apply to you. If not, see if you can write down some reasons that you *should* feel confident. This list can include your past achievements, and past successes. Surely, there are reasons that you should be confident. Think about the kinds of compliments that you hear about yourself from other people. Consider the things that you value most about yourself.

When it comes to weight loss, many people feel that they can only be confident after they have already achieved the perfect body they are looking for. After all, how could you be confident in advance of achieving your goals? The fact of the matter is that when you truly have faith that the Law of Attraction is bringing you the results that you are looking for, you can have advance confidence that you will soon be achieving your goals.

We definitely can be confident in our bodies. After all, your body knows how to be healthy and fit when you give it the right tools. Once you set the process in motion, your body will drop the pounds and give you the results you are seeking. Your body is your friend. Your body has innate knowledge about how to lose weight and become healthier.

In fact, when you gain weight, your body is just trying to do the right thing. The body often gains weight to seek to protect you, not to harm you. Fat actually has a reason that it exists! It often serves to store unhealthy substances that get into our system. Our bodies are just trying to protect us from what it deems is not healthy. However, just like your body gains weight to seek to protect you, give your body the proper tools and it will work steadily on your behalf to drop pounds and burn fat. You have this inner knowledge within you. You can be confident that your body will do the right thing.

Why Confidence is So Important for the Law of Attraction

In order to make the Law of Attraction work on your behalf, it is extremely important to have confidence both in yourself as well as in the process. Often people have a low level of confidence due to experiences that have occurred in their lives. Negative past events can be unfortunate, but you need to move past them and embrace your ability to succeed.

... it is extremely important to have confidence both in yourself as well as in the process.

Often when people are trying to lose weight, they are held back from the times in the past when they have not lost weight. Many people feel as though they can only be confident about losing weight if they have a history of success at losing weight. Obviously, this is a flawed assumption. If only people with a prior record of success could lose weight, then no one would be doing so. Surely, all the weight loss companies around the world would go out of business is *no one* was ever losing weight. Allow yourself to overcome the impulse to assume you will be unsuccessful. Millions of people have lost weight, and you can too.

When you aren't truly confident, you will see scenarios that have often occurred in the past occur again. Obviously, now is the time you have decided to lose weight and achieve a new fit, healthy body. You have outgrown the need for these past types of events. It is time to embrace something new. In order to achieve these goals, you also must embrace a new better and more confident you.

It is important to realize that whether or not you lost weight in the past is no longer relevant. Every day is new and past successes or failures no longer can hold any kind of dominion over you. When you are truly confident, it will radiate from your being. You will know that you will be a healthy weight soon, and others will know it as well.

Here are some items that may deter your confidence when you are trying to lose weight:

- **Negative Self-Talk**

  Many people, who have trouble attaining their desired weight, constantly berate themselves with negative self-talk. Often they may not even be aware that they are doing this. In order to boost your confidence, you must get rid of this kind of negativity in your life.

  Take a day where you do not permit yourself to say anything negative about yourself either out loud to others or to yourself. Try to make it through an entire day. When you have gotten through one day, you can try to see if you can get through two days. Eventually if you keep playing this game, you will see that you have managed to keep the negative self-talk at bay for a week or maybe even a month. You will find that in the process, you will grow more and more confident and happy.

  While you are at it, try to resist saying anything negative about anyone else in your life as well! You will find this to be a highly educational experience. Many people who try this experiment are amazed that on their first attempt that they often can't go more than a couple of hours without thinking something negative about themselves or someone else.

- **Residual Memories**

  If you have tried dieting in the past, and your weight loss did not go as well as expected, these memories can still be holding power over you in the present. They may keep you feeling depressed and unmotivated. Even if you haven't tried to drop pounds before, the experience of having failed in general could be having a negative impact on you right now.

  Lets face it; failing can be traumatic, especially when we are very young. Again, it is important to realize that every day is new, and the past does not have any control over you. Every day, you have the power to think new, fresh thoughts and have total control over the food and exercise that you partake in.

- **Memories From Childhood**

  Quite frequently people have negative, painful memories about being "fat" as a child. It is no secret that children who are overweight are frequently tormented and teased by their peers. Name-calling and insults can sometimes stay with people for a lifetime. If you were called cruel nicknames and received verbal abuse around the issue of your weight when you are young, it could be holding you back from achieving the positive results that you are seeking today.

  Now is the time to look at this situation objectively. Do you really think its right that something that an 8 year old said 20 or 30 years ago should be impacting your present life? Because if you are letting incidences of childhood bullying effect you now, you are indeed letting children from the past have dominion over your life. Believe it or not, there are 48-year-old grown men who are making decisions based on what an 8 year old told them 40 years ago. How can an 8 year old keep a 48 year old from attaining the level of health and fitness he desires? When you understand how little sense it makes to be held back by childhood memories, you will begin to make true progress towards your goal of health.

- **Parental Belief Systems**

  Often people do have their self-belief system past on to them by one or more parents. Think back for a moment. Did your mother or father constantly put him or herself down? Did you constantly hear one of them (or both of them) say "I can't do this," "I am not good enough to do that," and so on? If so, you may be modeling behavior from when you were just a child. However, realizing that this is what you are doing is the best way to move on and leave your own negativity and confidence problems behind you.

- **A Belief that You Constantly Fail at Things that You Try**

If you feel that you can't achieve your new desired weight because you constantly fail at things you do, you are not seeing the big picture. If you honestly believe this, you are definitely one of the people who see the glass half empty instead of half full. You need to release this habit of negative thinking.

Look around you and consider all that you have succeeded with in your life. Think about what you have overcome in your life to get to where you are today! You certainly have succeeded on numerous occasions in your life, and you have the ability to succeed at any goal you set including reaching your new desired weight.

- **Underlying Negative Ideas About One's Self**

Many people suffer from low self-esteem, and they believe that they actually don't deserve to be thin. If you think that this description fits you, it is time to let go of these subconscious beliefs. Positive affirmations and hypnosis can work wonders to help you get rid of these negative ideas about yourself. Remember that you are a good person, and you deserve all the best that life has to offer. You also deserve to have the healthiest and longest life possible.

- **Negative and Unsupportive People**

Often those around us determine so much of what we think and believe. If you realize that you need to improve your level of confidence, give some thought to the people that you typically interact with. Are these people supporting your growth and success?

Many success experts have commented that it is essential to surround yourself with people that you find inspirational and motivating. Particularly when you are seeking to make progress in your life, it is important to be sure to avoid people who are bringing you down. Zig Ziglar once said, "Life is too short to spend your precious time trying to convince a person who wants to live in gloom and doom otherwise. Give lifting that person your best shot, but don't hang around long enough for his or her bad attitude to pull you down. Instead, surround yourself with optimistic people."

- **Being Unsure of How to Get Healthy**

Sometimes people convince themselves that they can't lose weight because they just don't know how. They tell themselves they don't know how to cook healthy food, or that they don't know how to exercise. Of course, throw out these notions as they are silly and will not serve you. Even if you don't know how to make a gourmet healthy meal, there are plenty of simple easy foods that can be prepared in a matter of minutes. In fact, we will get into some of these recipes later on in this book.

As far as exercising goes, there is no advanced level exercise that must be achieved to lose weight. You also don't need to spend the money to hire a personal trainer or join a fancy gym. You can exercise every day and never spend a dime. After all, we have known how to walk or how to run for years. Walking, running, biking or swimming are all effective forms of exercise.

- **Comparing Yourself to Other People**

How many of us lose confidence by constantly comparing ourselves to others? This is a habit that most of us are guilty of at some point or another. In fact, many people get into a bad habit with comparisons early in life. Parents often set up a scenario where one child is living in the shadow of the other. They may say things like, "Why can't you be more like other kids?" or "Why can't you do better in school like your sister?"

Little do parents realize it at the time, but these kinds of statements can set a child up for a lifetime of comparing him or herself to other people. This kind of thinking makes many people feel as though they are never good enough. This can be a serious problem, especially when it comes to weight loss goals.

Make sure you stop comparing yourself to other people. Don't pick up magazines and compare yourself to models. If you find yourself watching a movie or TV show and comparing yourself to the actors or actresses, shift your thinking to something else. Now is the time for you to focus on yourself.

If you keep comparing yourself to others, you will never have the chance to truly improve your own life. Remember, many of these actors and models are also insecure about their own looks. Also many of them are airbrushed or "photoshopped" by magazine designers. You can never know the truth about other people, but you can know the truth about yourself.

- **You are Afraid of Change**

Often people can't move on and end up getting stuck in the past, simply because they are afraid of the new. Even if people aren't happy with their current situation, they often find it difficult to progress to the next chapter of their life. If you think this description suits you, just be sure to breathe, relax, and focus on welcoming the next chapter of your life.

Through mindfulness and using the Law of Attraction, each year is certain to be better than the last! Be excited about change and be sure to embrace it with open arms.

How to Keep Your Level of Confidence High

It is important to keep your confidence level high while you are attracting what you want in your life. After all, your thoughts create your reality. If you aren't 100% sure of how you feel or what you want, these thoughts will start to surface in your reality. Sometimes we can literally become our own worst enemy.

Lets get off the topic of weight loss for a moment. To make the point, lets focus on a topic like dating. Take the example of Molly. She meets a man named Chris and instantly becomes infatuated with him. She finally decides to ask him out on a date, and to her pleasant surprise, Chris says yes. Chris and Molly agree to meet at a certain time on Saturday at a nearby coffee shop.

On the day of the date, Molly becomes worried and nervous. Her lack of confidence begins to show through. She goes to her closet to pick out an outfit to wear on the date, and can't find anything that she feels makes her look good enough. She stands at her closet for over an hour obsessing over what she should wear. Suddenly, she looks at her watch and realizes she is now 30 minutes late. Molly quickly calls Chris' cell phone, he tells her that he has already left the coffee shop.

Chris is irritated as he was excited to meet up with Molly, but after 30 minutes waiting for her in the coffee shop, he came to the conclusion she stood him up. Chris says, "Maybe some other time," although he doesn't really mean it. He has sized Molly up as being too unreliable to date anyhow.

Do you see how in the scenario above Molly has sabotaged her own success due to lack of confidence? This same type of self-sabotage happens frequently to people in a wide variety of areas of their lives, career, relationships, weight loss, etc. While they are busy obsessing and worrying, a significant opportunity may fall through.

Think about when you were a student. When you went into a test thinking, "I am definitely going to fail" didn't you usually fail? Isn't a better choice to think that you will ace the test? Even if you failed countless tests in the past, that doesn't mean you will fail this time. When you walk into a test feeling confident, well-prepared and positive, your results on the test will always be better.

So what can we do to improve our levels of confidence? Here are some things you can try in your life to boost your confidence while achieving your weight loss goals:

- **Practice Hobbies or Activities That You Love**

  Truly, we are most confident when we are doing what we love. In the days when you are waiting for your weight loss goals to be achieved, try following up on new hobbies or old hobbies that make you feel good about yourself. Were you a high school tennis star? Perhaps join a club where you can play some tennis. Do you know that you have skill at painting? If so, start painting and let those positive confident feelings surge through you! Try to feel these same sorts of feelings when you are doing activities that are connected to your new body, such as exercising and making healthy food choices.

- **Tackle Small Things You Have een Meaning to Try**

  Often succeeding at small things in our lives can slowly build up our confidence. Also trying new things allows us to face our fears. When you go ahead and try new things that make you feel good, it is beneficial for building up your character too. Think of it like training. The more new things you try and succeed at, the more you will strengthen your "success muscles."

- **Ask Friends and Family What They Admire About You**

  Tell people you are losing weight and looking for a shot of self-confidence. Ask people if they could chime in with some positive words about you. You can even post on your facebook status, "Can someone say something nice about me today? I need a confidence booster." If you don't believe, it go ahead and try it as an experiment. Most likely, you will be overwhelmed with positive feedback. Don't be timid to ask for this type of input. After all, your friends know that you will give them back the same praise and admiration one day when they need it.

- **Explore New Things**

  When we explore things that are new, it can often be great for our confidence.

- **Help Other People**

  Another great way to build up your confidence is to volunteer or do something concrete that helps other people. Of course, this is a good thing to do in general no matter what your goals are. Plus when you give to others, you always receive something back. And you will also see the valuable difference that you can quickly make in someone else's life.

- **Set Daily Goals and Achieve Them**

  Setting small goals and achieving them is a great way to build up your comfort level with success. For example, you can tell yourself that you will eat an apple every day on your diet, and achieve that goal. Or you can tell yourself every morning you will sit and meditate for five minutes before getting out of bed. This is another goal that can be easily met and achieved.

  Every time you succeed at one of these "mini goals" give yourself a pat on the back. Really take time to appreciate the fact that you set out a goal and achieved it. Try to bask in the feeling of success for a few minutes before you go throughout your day.

- **Read More Books**

There are plenty of books on the topic of confidence and overcoming fear. A classic on this topic is *Feel the Fear and Do it Anyway.* If you read books about how other people have become more confident, you can begin to change your behavior to be more like theirs.

- **Watch Inspiring Films**

If you are feeling your confidence level is weak, why not take the time to watch an inspiring film? If you can't think of any inspiring films, simply take a moment and search "inspiring films" on Google. We guarantee that some new selections you have never even heard of will pop up in your search.

- **Use Self-Hypnosis and Auto-Suggestion to Build Confidence**

If you make the commitment to turn the corner on your level of confidence through self-hypnosis, it can make a huge difference. You can just listen to a mp3 at night before you go to bed. Steve's website even has hypnosis audio that you can listen to as you go throughout your day called Daytime Recordings. Gradually, new positive ones will replace your negative unconfident thoughts. You can find self-hypnosis audio that is specifically geared to improve your confidence.

If you don't feel like buying hypnosis mp3s to gain more confidence, you can also try self-affirmation. Affirmations are free, and you can stand in the mirror and read them to yourself any time of day. With an affirmation, you simply need to repeat a positive statement over and over to yourself. It can be something very simple like "I possess infinite confidence." You can do this in the morning and in the evening. In fact, the more times a day you can repeat affirmations to yourself, the better.

Here is a sample script for becoming more confident. This is something that is extremely helpful to read several times, perhaps at the beginning of the day. If you are craving dessert or struggling to make a good food choice, you can also stop and read though this script.

I am supremely confident. Whether or not I have failed in the past is unimportant. The important thing is that I am confident now. I am comfortable with any situation that comes my way. I am constantly admiring all of my wonderful qualities. I am an amazing human being! I accept myself thoroughly no matter what weight I am at. I am breathing in and out deeply. With every breath I inhale, I am becoming more confident and powerful. With ever breath I exhale, I am letting go of my fear and lack of confidence from the past. It is so easy to lose weight and achieve the perfect body that

I was born to have. I have everything I need at my disposal in order to lose weight or be successful at everything that I try. I remember plenty of times in my life that I was completely confident and totally successful. My weight loss journey is just like this past example of success. I am so lucky to be free of the weight that I have been carrying. I am becoming a more confident, successful and peaceful individual every day.

Chapter 5

FOOD CHOICES

"He who takes medicine and neglects diet,
wastes the skill of the physicians." —Chinese Proverb

Now that you are using the Law of Attraction to create a new slimmer you, it is time to really hone in on what foods your body wants. Part of what causes the Law of Attraction to work in the first place is your vibrational energy. Our bodies are vibrating right along with the rest of the universe. When your vibration is higher, the things that you want in your life will come to you even quicker. This fact is not just true for attracting your new body, but it also is the case for anything new that you want to bring into your life.

When you truly understand the importance of your vibrational energy, you will realize that your food choices have a big effect on how you feel and the vibrations that you are sending out to the universe. Haven't you noticed how your food and energy level can change depending on what you eat?

Think about the difference in how you feel when you drink a cup of chamomile tea versus a can of soda. While the tea may help you feel calm and relaxed, the soda will undoubtedly make you feel jittery and restless. Similarly, your energy will feel differently when you eat a simple piece of fruit like an apple versus something on the other end of the spectrum that is highly processed like a frozen pizza. You are constantly changing your energy level by what you choose to eat. Therefore, how you feel every day and your ability to most effectively use the Law of Attraction for your own benefit is influenced by your food choices.

It is time to treat your body like the temple that it is. Yes, we have all heard the saying "your body is a temple." Perhaps this statement sounds clichéd at this point;

41

however, it is still true. If your body is buzzing with positive energy from nutritious fruits and vegetables, you will actually have an easier time achieving and creating all that you want in your life.

Also it is important to note that some foods have been proven to actually cause negative emotions. We will explore this topic and what foods to avoid more in the upcoming chapter "10 Foods You Should Never Eat Again." However, it is important to point out that food can raise or lower your energy quite rapidly. Your food choices have an amazing power over your life. Food has tremendous ability to either harm us or heal us, depending on what we choose.

> Your food choices have an amazing power over your life.

Listen to the Food Choices that Your Body Wants

When you are shopping in the grocery store, pay attention to what sections of the store you gravitate to. Are these the aisles of the grocery store that will have the best impact on your health and vibrational level? Also ask yourself if there are items that you are reaching for at the store strictly out of habit. Many people develop bad eating habits throughout life, and then just don't think to change these habits. For example, maybe you have started your day by eating sugary breakfast cereal since you were a kid. Without giving it any thought, you might be still tossing the same cereal into your shopping cart.

If you are still going down the aisle and choosing sugary cereal for breakfast even though you are an adult, it is time to stop and take a look at this choice. Sure the cereal might taste good, and it is what you are used to eating, but is it really the best choice you can make? Now is the time to take an honest look at what you eat and reassess if you are really making the best choices for your health. Just because you are directed to a certain food out of habit doesn't mean that you instinctively want it.

It is important to stop looking at food strictly evaluating calories and fat. When you do this, you can often overlook foods that your body needs and craves simply because it is high fat. For example, an avocado is full of fat, but has the kind of fat your body needs. A highly processed cookie that is claiming to be low-fat and low-calorie, however, may be exactly the kind of food that you don't need. Even though this cookie will fit into your daily allotment of calories, it is not providing your body with the nutrition it requires. There is definitely a difference between good calories and bad calories.

Start Approaching Food Intentionally

Lets say that you are in the cookies/cracker aisle, and you are about to put a big bag of cookies into your cart. Here are some examples of questions that you could stop and ask yourself.

1. What will the experience of eating these cookies really be like?

    Sure, they will taste delicious and crunchy at first. But what will the experience of eating these cookies *really* be like? Sugar usually gives us a quick high, but then just as quickly as it brings us up, it brings us lows. Sugar lows can include depression, irritation, anger, and fatigue, to name just a few emotions.

2. Do these cookies truly serve my needs?

    Sure the cookies will taste good for a few minutes as you eat them, but do they truly serve your needs? Take a minute and think of what your needs are. You want to not only achieve your goals of dropping pounds, but you also want to make sure all of the cells in your body are optimally functioning.

3. Are these cookies supporting my body nutritionally?

    Your body has certain important nutritional requirements. When we choose what we eat every day, we need to make sure we are giving our body all the nutrition that it needs. After all, our body works hard serving us every day doing things like pumping our blood, eliminating waste and allowing our heart to beat, shouldn't we return the favor to our body? Shouldn't we enable it to get the best nutrition possible?

    Take a look at the ingredient list in the cookies. If there are ingredients on the list that you don't understand or can't pronounce, how can you be confident that your body will know how to process this ingredient? If you don't know what the ingredient actually is, do you really think it is likely to be supporting your nutritional needs?

4. Are these cookies in line with my highest good?

    There are a variety of things in your life that feed (literally) your higher good. These can include everything under the sun and will vary from person to person. Examples of what might be in line with your highest good include things like meditation, yoga, spending time with friends, hiking, drinking water, and so on. Now ask yourself, are eating these cookies in line with your highest good?

5. Can I make a better decision right now?

    Every moment you do have the opportunity to make whatever decision you feel is most empowering for you. Now look at the bag and cookies and ask yourself if you could make a better decision.

Once you start asking yourself these types of questions when you go shopping, you will slowly alter what food choices you want to make. Eventually instead of taking time to ask yourself these questions every time you are at the grocery store, healthy and productive thoughts will come to you automatically. Your body, mind and spirit will instantly give you the necessary feedback if you should be eating the cookies or whatever else you are considering putting in your shopping cart.

Eating Intuitively

Take yourself to the produce aisle of the grocery store and see how the foods strike you. Don't just pass them by quickly. Take time to contemplate the different fruits and vegetables and how they might feel in your body. Appreciate the variety of colors, shapes and sizes of the food that nature provides. Isn't it amazing that these foods are exactly the ones that offer antioxidants, vitamins and minerals for your body?

Take a piece of fruit and go ahead and ask yourself the same 5 questions as you asked about the cookies. Lets take for example, a pear.

1.   What will the experience of eating this pear really be like?

     The pear will be juicy, naturally sweet, and crunchy. Parts of the pear may even be soft and tender. After eating the pear, very likely I will feel energetic and happy. I do not foresee any negative impact from eating this pear.

2.   Does this pear truly serve my needs?

     Yes, in fact it does. A pear will fit in nicely with my current agenda of dropping some weight. In fact, pears are great for weight loss. One pear has about 98 calories.

3.   Will this pear support my body nutritionally?

     Yes, definitely. Pears have a high amount of Vitamin C, Vitamin K and dietary fiber. Pears also have copper, which can protect us from free radical damage.

4.   Is this pear in line with my highest good?

     Yes.

5.   Can I make a better decision right now?

     The pear seems to be a great decision.

Eat with the Seasons, Eat Local

One way to really get in touch with your ability to eat intuitively is to go to farmers markets and see firsthand what food are in season. What foods are being grown locally right in your community? When you stroll along in a farmer's market, you can see the foods right along with the people who actually grow these foods. When you see food in this setting, you quickly are reminded how amazing it is that this delicious bounty was actually grown from the earth. Often in the grocery store, we lose touch with what we are really eating and the origins of our food.

Plus, even when we do choose healthy foods, they can come from the other side of the globe. During transportation, foods can lose some of their nutritional content. Fresh foods that were recently just in the earth have a higher nutritional density. This means more availability of nutritional elements for your body. Another benefit to eating food from a farmer's market is that you are supporting the local farmers in your area. Many small farms can go out of business due to lack of money. When you give money directly to the farmers, it encourages them to keep providing healthy food for you and the rest of your community.

Make Sure you are Eating Whole Foods

Another important aspect to food choices is to make sure that you are eating whole foods. Sure, chemical laced foods packed with preservatives may taste good at the moment, but they will do little to help you reach your goals. When you eat whole foods, you will find that they can be just as delicious and satisfying as junk food. We also recommend buying food that is labeled organic.

So what are whole foods? These are foods that are as close to their natural form as possible. They do not contain added ingredients, like colorings, fat or preservatives. Eating raw fruits and vegetables are some of the best ways to get whole foods into your diet. When you eat whole foods you are getting food the way nature intended. Therefore, it is easier for your body to utilize this food in a beneficial manner. Often when foods are processed, vital nutritional elements are removed. Even worse, is that usually when food is processed, bad things are added in. When manufacturers process foods, it is easy for them to add things like preservatives, food colorings, and high levels of salt and sugar. These are all things that your body does not want or need.

Good whole foods selections include nuts and seeds, beans, milk, eggs, meat, poultry and fish. However, remember, in order for something to be a "whole food" it must not be processed. Therefore, something like a hot dog, or meat lasagna from the frozen food section of the grocery store would no longer be considered a whole food. We will get more into ideas for whole foods recipes in the third part of this book.

Creating a Vision Board

If you are struggling making the best food choices, one very useful idea is to create a vision board. This process will support your goals for the new weight that you will be manifesting. Visualization is a very important part of getting the Law of Attraction to work for your benefit. A vision board will help you visualize because it gives you something concrete to create and look at when you are working on focusing on what you want to create in your life.

A vision board is a place to collect all of your ideas for your hopes and dreams. You can also use a book or album for your visions. Simply find photos or images that are symbolic of what you want to achieve. So when it come to creating a vision board to inspire you to make the proper food choices, feel free to find gorgeous images of fresh fruit, colorful vegetables or whatever else you want to eat more of to support your health and fitness goals.

While you are at it, you can also add whatever other images seem suitable and exciting to you when you think of your goals. All of these images should bring you a sense of exhilaration. Hopefully, if you do this exercise correctly, when you look at the vision board your pulse will race a little and you will feel instantly happier.

So in the spirit of your health and fitness goals, you could put images including things like the Hawaiian island where you will vacation in your new bikini, the new dress that you will buy as soon as you reach your intended goal, the mountains you will be hiking as you achieve your goals of radiant health, the list can go on and on. Truly, this is a personal exercise so the visions that get you motivated are ones that are very much personal to you.

Along with your images, go ahead and put text in that inspires you to make the proper food choices too. The text can be phrases motivating you to exercise, stay on track, be persistent, or whatever else makes you feel confident and powerful. Again the text should be very personal to you. Don't be generic. Your vision board should really only be effective to you, don't gear it to be read by other people.

When you set out to create your vision board, try to get into the spirit of being childlike and innocent. Try to get back to the time before you had formed notions of what is possible and impossible. As we get older, we often start to get way too attached to a voice in our head that controls what we think is logical or not logical. In other words, it is easy to get jaded. For the purposes of creating the vision board, it is important to try to get back to that time before you instantly decided what was possible or not. You should feel as though all paths are open and ready for you to embark upon them.

When you create this vision board, remember that you should be having a blast. After all, you are honing in on the things that will be bringing you happiness and joy in the future. If you find that you aren't feeling happy and excited when creating your vision board, take a break and get back to it later. For the purpose of the exercise, this activity should make you feel hopeful and optimistic. If you are getting stressed out and worrying about what you have or have not already achieved, try getting back to the vision board another day when you are in a better state of mind.

Remember in our Confidence chapter how we discussed the many things that impact us in childhood that now lead to our belief structures about whether or not we can succeed. These are exactly the types of feelings that you should try to overcome while creating your vision board. Who cares if you feel silly putting the board together? The bottom line is that a vision board works when it comes to manifesting your hopes and dreams. It only makes sense for you to take advantage of that fact and to use one in your life.

Once you have your vision board, you can keep it in a place where you will see it frequently. If your vision board ends up being really geared towards food choices, why not go ahead and post it right on the refrigerator? Having your inspirational words and motivational images staring at you right on the fridge can do wonders to guide you to eat the foods that are in line with your highest intentions.

Plan Ahead

One of the most important habits you can get into for sustaining your new health and fitness is to plan ahead. You may even start planning out weekly menus. It is a great idea to make meals ahead of time and freeze them so that you have them on hand later when you are busy. This is a great trick that works perfectly when you are making big soups or vegetable dishes.

Another trick is to never be caught in a situation where you would potentially need to turn to a fast food counter or a twinkie. Keep healthy foods around so that you always have a back-up option that is healthy. You can keep a bag of nuts or trail mix around in the glove compartment of the car, for example. This simple easy idea will help you from visiting the fast food chains when you are driving in your car. If hunger strikes, you can simply pull a nutritious snack out that you have left for yourself. Again, just remember to plan ahead. This means when you are running low on nuts, just replace your stash.

Another great idea is to keep fresh fruit around at work. Having fruit available will prevent you from going to the vending machine or eating candy that might be around at your workplace. Some companies even hire a fruit at work delivery service to deliver fresh fruit directly to the workplace. This kind of service is a great idea because it saves people the hassle of going to the store, picking out fruit, and then remembering to take it to work. Perhaps see if a few coworkers want to go in on ordering this fruit together. You probably will have more and more people eager to chip in and join you once they see the convenience of the fresh fruit showing up at the door.

Some other good ideas for foods to have around include the following:

- Dried Fruit
- Nuts and seeds
- Fresh chopped veggies
- Trail mix
- Healthy sugar free organic muffins
- Fresh fruit juice
- Vegetable juice
- Organic sugar free nutrition bars

Learn to Cook

Many people have found that if they want to enjoy a wide variety of foods and also keep the weight off, a great idea is to learn to cook. When you can cook at home, you know exactly what is going into your food. Plus, you are less tempted to eat enticing things that are presented to you at a restaurant like bread, sodas and desserts. You also can keep an eye on how many calories are going into your meals.

> When you can cook at home, you know exactly what is going into your food.

Here is another problem with restaurants that you have undoubtedly noticed. These days, massive portion sizes are all too common, especially in the U.S. When you are out eating and socializing with friends, it is easy to just keep eating and eating. When there is a huge amount of food on your plate, it is difficult to know how much food your body actually wants or needs. On the other hand, when you cook at home, you can give yourself the proper sized portion and go back for seconds if you are still hungry.

There are other benefits to cooking too. You certainly can save money by preparing your own meals. Everyone knows that going out to dinner (and even frequently going for fast food) can certainly add up and put a toll on your budget.

Cooking is also a fun activity for you and your significant other or for you and your family. And if you are dating, there is really nothing like impressing your date with a home cooked meal that you made. You can experiment with the wide variety of cuisines from around the world that offer healthy foods.

Slow Food Movement

One recent organization that has helped a lot of people reconnect with the pleasures associated with food is the Slow Food movement. Slow Food encourages us to slow down and enjoy our food. The organization was founded in 1989 with the stated mission "to counteract fast food and fast life, the disappearance of local food traditions and people's dwindling interest in the food they eat, where it comes from, how it tastes and how our food choices affect the rest of the world." Slow Food also emphasizes protecting biodiversity and local farmers.

This organization syncs up with quite a few of the concepts around eating we stressing in this book. The movement encourages people to eat slowly and enjoy their food. This is a great thing for you to keep in mind when you are seeking to continue your diet. In order to properly digest your food, it is important not to rush. When you eat too quickly we consume calories before our body is even able to catch up and understand what has happened. People generally end up eating fewer calories when they eat slowly.

Chapter 6

STOP BINGE EATING

"We never repent of having eaten too little ." —Thomas Jefferson

There are various levels of binge eating. As a result, the term "binge eating" can have a variety of meanings. On one level, binge eating can be a serious eating disorder where people actually overeat to the point where they cannot stop eating. However, many people will reference that they have been "binge eating" when in fact they have merely been overeating every now and then. Occasional binge eating can be more thought of as severe straying off your diet or "falling off the wagon."

Before we begin, it is very important to note that very severe binge eating is quite serious, and it is often an issue that requires medical attention. There are a variety of medical professionals that are trained to deal with binge eating when it is actually an eating disorder. If you are suffering from an eating disorder, please realize that you can most certainly find help and stop binge eating. People do so every single day and there is no reason you cannot and will not join their ranks!

In short, binge eating is when people simply eat uncontrollably. For those who are seeking to lose weight and have a healthy lifestyle, binge eating simply does not fit in any way, shape or form. Yet you should not feel alone if you are binge eating. Estimates indicate that between two and three percent of the population binge eats in some fashion or another.

In fact, Harvard Medical School recently did a study that stated that 3.5% of women and 2% of men are binge eaters. Clearly, this is a lot of people. Here is an idea to give you an idea of how many people this is. Just

... 3.5% of women and 2% of men are binge eaters.

imagine if tomorrow you woke up and the news was all abuzz with the fact that between two and three percent of the population went on a hunger strike. That would certainly get your attention, wouldn't it? So you should never feel alone if you do suffer from this particular eating disorder.

How To Deal With Binge Eating

It is very common for those who suffer from binge eating to feel depressed either during or after the period during which they are binge eating. Like most eating disorders, binge eating usually occurs in private. This indicates that those sufferers uncomfortable or ashamed of acknowledging their disorder. It is common sense that being ashamed of any disorder can make it more difficult for one to seek and find treatment. Treatments vary on a case-by-case basis, but through working with medical professionals such as doctors, psychiatrists and nutritionists it is possible to make great strides in treating binge eating.

So how do you know if your binge eating is technically an eating disorder? Those with an eating disorder will typically eat a large amount of food in a short period of time at least twice a week. If you are binge eating only occasionally, once a month or every few months, then you have an overeating problem, but not necessarily an eating disorder.

Hypnotism can also do wonders to treat binge eating. Steve has had massive success with many clients who have cured their binge eating forever under his guidance. Steve also has a very effective self-hypnosis CD and MP3 that has helped many people overcome binge eating. The techniques in these hypnosis materials target the emotional stress that causes binge eating.

When you are using the Law of Attraction to guide you towards your goal of being healthy, it is critical that you make a firm decision you no longer want to experience periods of binge eating. Others, such as medical professionals or friends and family, might help you along the way or give you a strong push to get and receive help.

However, ultimate success and happiness will depend upon you and deciding what you want and what you don't want. Consider this fact for a moment, your friends and family or doctor will not be with you at three fifteen in the morning when you decide to binge eat. You are the only one that can keep you from binge eating in the end.

There is little chance of stopping binge eating without first tapping into and understanding why you are binge eating. Often people who do not address other issues and problems in their life end up binge eating. Food, and the abuse of food, is used to cover up or mask other problems that they may be experiencing. Thus, emotional problems are often at the core of binge eating. If you are binge eating, it may be helpful to stop and simply ask yourself why you are doing so. Once you have uncovered the root of the problem, it may be easier to get beyond it.

Emotional Responses and Binge Eating

Using the Law of Attraction to eliminate your binge eating for good will work much better if you also know what triggers you. You might be going about your day and suddenly without warning you beginning eating and you simply do not stop. Perhaps you were thinking about something stressful or traumatic, or perhaps something happened that "set you off."

Imagine that you pass a mean, aggressive barking dog on your way home from work. Perhaps you immediately go home, start eating and don't stop for several hours. This series of events would seem to indicate that the barking dog, or something about the environment of stress that was created by the barking dog, served as a trigger. Something about the barking dog triggered the emotions that led to binge eating. The key word here is emotion.

For most people, binge eating is triggered by emotional responses. Next time you feel like binge eating, instead of going straight to the refrigerator or to the drive-thru, sit down for a moment. Perhaps pour yourself a glass of water or make yourself some tea. Now ask yourself what happened that day that might have triggered you. At first, nothing may come to mind.

Keep contemplating your day and what events occurred until you can identify your trigger. Who did you talk to? Where did you go? Did something different or new happen that bothered you? Once you know your trigger, you are already halfway towards unlocking the puzzle of why you binge eat.

If you can't figure out what may have triggered you, don't worry. Your emotional triggers may become clearer over time. For now, just try to be mindful of when and why you feel like binging. Generally binge eating is not caused by hunger, its caused by something else much deeper. Try to acknowledge that you may be covering up emotions through your eating patterns.

Overeating, How Were These Patterns Formed?

It only makes sense for us to explore why binge eating occurs. Perhaps you have had a stressful day and you just want to set down and get the pleasure rush from food. This is very common. At some point, virtually everyone has used food in this fashion. Food tastes good and it can instantly lift our spirits.

So what were the patterns that led to this overeating? Obviously, one issue is using food as a crutch for when we feel stressed in some way. It may be that we are feeling lonely, overworked or feeling as though we have failed at our diet. Anyone who has struggled with weight issues knows that it can be tempting to simply give up and eat.

Another pattern that can cause one to overeat is giving in to the feeling of denial. If you feel as though you have denied yourself pleasurable foods for too long, it can break your willpower. The end result is that you might just chow down and completely abandon your diet. One way to guard against this is to make sure that you are consistently focusing on positive intentions and actions as opposed to negative ones.

You want to make sure that you are eating enough calories and that your diet includes quality fats. You also want to make sure that you are enjoying the food that you are eating. If you feel as though everything you eat is a dry, unfulfilling rice cake, then you will be more likely to binge so that you can again derive some pleasure out of eating.

What to Do When You Feel Like Binging?

Visualizing is great way of using the Law of Attraction to your advantage. If you feel that your willpower might be slipping, simply take a moment out and shut your eyes. Now imagine how good you will feel when the day comes that you have achieved your perfect weight and are radiantly healthy. Imagine how much more confidence you will have. Imagine the feeling of satisfaction and happiness that this feeling will bring you.

Visualizing what you want is an important part of turning your dreams into a reality. In this specific case, your dream, the one you wish to turn into reality, is to achieve your perfect weight and be healthy. It is also important to state that you should be visualizing staying and *remaining* healthy. This means that you should be visualizing modifying your attitude towards food and your lifestyle in a positive manner. In this fashion, the universe can truly give you what you want, and that is to be healthy for good!

When you feel like overeating, visualize how your life will change. This type of visualization, of course, is tied to visualizing how you will feel when you are your perfect weight. But feel free to take it a step further and see how this new body and health will impact all areas of your life.

When you are feeling like you need to overeat and want to "take a break from your diet," visualize how your life will change once you have lost the weight. Visualize everything about how your life will change. Here are some ideas to help guide you in terms of what you can focus on and visualize when you are thinking about overeating.

Visualization Points For When You Feel Like Overeating

1. Visualize how you will look.
2. Visualize the new clothing you can now wear.
3. Visualize the reaction of your friends and family.
4. Visualize exciting activities that you will now do that you did not do before. There is likely something that you are not doing now that you would do if you were thinner and healthier.
5. Imagine the satisfaction and confidence you will have if you are able to successfully lose the weight and kept it off.

In short, if you are feeling like overeating and feel yourself giving in, just stop for a moment and visualize what your life could be like if you accomplish your goal. Constantly focusing on that goal, in this case dropping pounds and becoming healthier, will greatly increase your odds of success. Visualization will lead to focus. That focus will help you to lose the weight and keep the weight off. Just keep thinking about how your life will change when you lose the weight for good. Your emotions are so powerful. When they are used to your benefit, they can definitely assist you in overcoming your temptation to binge.

Other Strategies For Addressing Overeating

One major factor in overeating is a sense of denial. As we have covered earlier, feeling that you haven't had a favorite food or meal in a long time and begin to wreck havoc on any diet. Superhuman willpower is a pretty rare thing, and this means that you need to make sure that you avoid your breaking point. Visualizing yourself being thin will no doubt help you achieve your goals, but the proper strategy can also decrease the amount of pressure that you put on yourself. Here are a few strategies that you can employ to make sure that your resolve does not slip.

Ten Tips For Avoiding Overeating

1. Make sure that you have plenty of nutrition in your diet. Often when your body begins craving foods, it's simply due to the fact that you are feeling depleted due to lack of proper nutrition. Giving your body what it needs to function properly will help keep those pesky cravings at bay.

2. Find dessert recipes that are nutritious and low calorie. Learn several different kinds of desserts that you know how to make. Being able to satisfy your sweet tooth without abandoning your diet is a step in the right direction.

3. Now that you have a group of awesome low calorie and nutritious desserts, make sure that you keep some on hand and ready to eat. This does mean that you will have to resist the temptation to eat them. However, if you feel that your resolve is breaking and you are ready to abandon your diet, they sure will come in handy.

4. Having someone you can call when you think you might be getting ready to overeat is a very, very good idea. Knowing that you have a support system is a fine way to help guard against binging.

5. Realize that many foods, such as sugar, have addictive properties. Simply knowing this can clue you in to how you may need to modify your behavior in order to "stay on track."

6. Eating and boredom can definitely go hand in hand. This means that you need to make sure that you have plenty to keep you from getting bored or feeling lonely. Even if you have not traditionally been a "pet person," consider getting a pet to keep you company. Simply having the companionship may do wonders to head off any episodes of overeating.

7. It is also possible, of course, to have too much companionship. If you have a house full of kids, and friends and relatives constantly flowing in and out of your house, you may feel as though you don't have any time to yourself. When this happens you may feel like overeating for the pleasure of it. One good way to combat these feeling is to spend some private time alone in a place that is free of food.

8. Private time in general is a way to address the issue of binging. Taking fifteen or twenty minutes a day to meditate will help you stay calmer and more focused. Numerous medical studies and university studies around the world have shown that there are long-term health benefits from meditation. Thus, by meditating you can help prevent episodes of overeating and enjoy the medical benefits that mediation offers, such as the lowering of stress hormones such as cortisol.

9. Dining out can definitely be a serious opportunity for overeating. A great deal of social life can revolve around food and drink. Realizing this fact is important and planning for it ahead of time is critical. Try and plan in advance and look for restaurants that have good low-calorie options. Just remember that recent studies show that restaurants are understating the calories in their food, when they post them or make them public at least. With this important fact in mind, consider adding ten percent to twenty percent to any calorie number a restaurant might give you.

10. Drinking out with the boys, or girls, maybe fun but it can really hurt your diet. All those drinks whether they are pretty ones with umbrellas in them or even a good old-fashion manly beer, have calories. Often they have more calories than you think. Drinking is a very dangerous form of overeating, because you can be going off your diet in a major fashion without being aware of it.

11. Try self-hypnosis. This technique, of course, is highly recommended by us. It can do wonders to help you deal with the feelings that you need to binge.

Stopping Binge Eating for Good

Below we have enclosed a sample self-hypnosis script you can try. If you are feeling as though you need to binge eat, why not take out this script and read through it. These types of affirmations can be truly transformative.

Continue to relax and let go of stressful thoughts and feeling concerned what you should or should not be eating. Instead turn your focus to what kinds of foods are most beneficial for your body, mind and spirit. You will soon realize just how powerful you are and you realize just how much self-control you have. You are a powerful person with a tremendous amount of self-control. And you allow yourself to change negative eating patterns into a positive relationship with food and you allow this to take place easily and effortlessly. You are so very relaxed. And you find that you eat very small portions of food when you are hungry. You imagine your body to be like a furnace and you realize that you must keep that fire burning at a constant level, giving yourself an appropriate amount of energy in the form of food throughout your day. And so you keep the furnace stoked. And you are relaxed. You eat appropriate amounts of food when you are hungry and once you have eaten the appropriate amount of food you simply stop eating, you stop eating. And you realize that you are very comfortable eating small amounts of food on a regular basis, small amounts of food on a regular basis because you are relaxed and at ease. And if at any time you should feel any urge to go beyond a small amount of food, you should deal with the issue that causes those feelings, you deal with that issue in a very straightforward, direct, and mature way. And then you continue to relax and day by day you are becoming better and better at dealing with issues in your life. You see them as challenges which you will overcome. And so when you think of food you only think of eating food for energy. And you eat small amounts of food when you are hungry. And you relax between meals and you relax now deeper and deeper.

Final Thoughts

There are a great many ways that you can deal with the issue of binge eating. The first step is to realize that you must plan to deal with this issue head on. It is not a problem that you can simply ignore and not plan for. Left unchecked, binge eating can get more and more out of control. It can really take its toll on your health goals as well as your self-esteem.

Whether your binge eating qualifies as an eating disorder or not, you simply must have a plan to deal with binge eating. If left unchecked, binge eating is unlikely to go away all on by itself. Your positive intentions and actions, however, can cure binge eating for good. As outlined in this chapter, it is possible to think through ahead of time what you can do to make sure that binge eating is less likely to happen.

The simple act of reading this chapter and thinking about the points it raises, means that have taken a powerful and important step in the right direction. However, remember, if you are indeed binge eating more than twice a week, you should consider getting some professional help you get out of this situation in an even more immediate fashion.

You now have the tools you need to use the Law of Attraction to visualize your success. Focusing and concentrating on the dream of a healthy weight and losing your weight permanently is now in reach. Achieving a healthy weight and keeping to that weight is far from impossible. Remember that people do it everyday.

By adopting a program designed to prevent binge eating, such as outlined in the Ten Tips For Avoiding Overeating, you are greatly increasing your chances of success. Treat your weight loss and health goals like you would a job search, for example. You should formulate a strategy and then take the steps necessary to make sure that you will achieve your goals.

Don't be afraid to embrace notions and ideas that may differ from your comfort zone or that may feel awkward at first. The real trick is to embrace whatever works. Simple steps such as having healthy treats on hand are likely to go a long way. You will also find that when you start filling your body with whole foods and nutrients that it needs, you will be less likely to feel like binge eating in the first place.

Many of us eat when we are stressed. This means that anything you can do to avoid stress is good. Don't underestimate the detrimental nature of stress either. As it turns out, stress hormones such as cortisol work to age your body and they can do it quite rapidly. Taking steps to keep your stress levels low will not only translate into a healthier you, but one that is less likely to binge.

As most dieters know, the downward spiral of overeating can be a loop that (literally) feeds on itself endlessly. But by adopting the right tactics and strategies it will be possible for you to avoid binging, to stay focused and to visualize your weight loss. Remember visualizing that you can achieve radiant health is the key and most important step of all.

Chapter 7
EXERCISE (FOCUS ON MOTIVATION)

"You have brains in your head. You have feet in your shoes.
You can steer yourself in any direction you choose." —Dr. Seuss

Do you feel as though you just can't get motivated to exercise? If so, you definitely are not alone. Between work, hobbies, family, and just day-to-day life, many people find that there is very little time left to exercise. With that time, they just want to relax rather than start exercising. But let's not judge others or ourselves harshly. At the end of a busy day, it can be difficult to work out at home, let alone go to the gym. However, for those looking to drop pounds, burn fat, and get into shape, it is necessary to get motivated.

Essentially, we can use many of the same Law of Attraction techniques we use for other purposes to get our workout regimen on track as well. Don't focus on how difficult it is to exercise. Don't focus your lack of motivation. Of course, as we have discussed, if we focus on these elements, we will receive more of them due to "like attracts like."

If you focus on how unmotivated you are feeling, you will quickly find yourself feeling more and more unmotivated. On the other hand, if you feel unmotivated, but agree to go over your list of why you want to achieve a healthier weight, you will begin to feel your spirits lift. Once you get your body into motion, you will likely feel like staying in motion. The old principle of Newtonian physics, "A body in motion stays in motion…a body at rest stays at rest" definitely applies here! However, sometimes even contemplating what we want isn't enough to get oneself off of the sofa and into the gym. This chapter was written to explore what else we can do to get motivated to exercise.

The facts are that the human body was designed to be used and to exercise. While many of us may spend our days behind desks moving paper, staring at computer screens or sitting in a car, that is not what the human body was designed to do. With this in mind, realize that you were meant to be active; you were meant to be running, walking and lifting objects. It's only in the last few decades that our collective level of physical activity has begun to slip a bit. Don't let this modern shift in physical activity confuse you. You were built from the DNA up to engage in physical activity. Once you have broken your old patterns you will indeed crave that physical activity!

One big important step is to focus what you do love about exercise. Now, many people will read this sentence and think to themselves, "What I really love about exercise? Just about nothing!" However, when you really break it down, most people can think of *something* that they love about exercising. And most people will find some forms of exercise more fun and joyous than others.

For example, you may hate jogging, but going rock climbing sounds fun to you. Or perhaps you despise going to the gym, but you love getting outdoors and hiking. Try to open your mind to all forms of exercise and which forms may appeal to you. Your new favorite sport or activity may be something you have not even tried yet!

> ... open your mind to all forms of exercise and which forms may appeal to you.

Letting Go of Making Excuses

It is easy to say that you don't have time to exercise, but in actuality, exercising doesn't have to be something that takes you all day or even hours. Just taking a brief amount of time out to move your body can be helpful. The body was designed to move. If you lead a sedentary lifestyle, you just won't look or feel your best. After all, we were designed to be physical creatures and not just sit in a cubicle all day with no sunshine. We are not meant to spend our time just watching television.

Remember that exercise can cause a massive boost to endorphin levels. In this way, it will complement your Law of Attraction work. If you exercise consistently, you will constantly have endorphins in your body that will help you stay positive, happy and ready to manifest what you want via the Law of Attraction.

Many people come up with an endless sea of excuses to keep them from having to go exercise. Using the Law of Attraction you should be able to overcome any or all excuses that could come up. Think of yourself as a creative machine that can overcome any problem. Once you shift your thinking, you will quickly see that you can come up with solutions to most problems.

For example, do you tell yourself that you can't workout because you cannot afford it? If you do, why not try running? Running is a great form of cardio exercise. You can start off slow and increase your endurance and how far you go. Running is also a great way to get fresh air and sunlight. It also gives you a chance to get out and visit new areas of your city or town. Why not take a short drive to a new part of town? When you get out of the car and take your jog, you can explore a whole new part of town you may not be familiar with. You may find great new restaurants, coffee shops and neighborhoods along the way. Many athletes also love running up and down hills. Again this is a great exercise that is also free. Running up hills can burn a lot of calories; it can also really give you great leg muscles.

Another great free form of exercise is biking. Just like running, biking allows you to get outside and see new areas. Once people get out on the road on a bicycle, they actually start to get addicted to this mode of transportation. Before they know it, they are taking their bike out to go and do errands.

In addition to being great for your legs, biking is also great for your core muscles, your abdominal area and back. Strengthening your core muscles will give you added strength to do many day-to-day activities. People who have switched to commuting to and from work on a bike as opposed to a car have been shown to lose weight, even while eating the same things. It is a great way to naturally get exercise into your day-to-day routine.

Besides just the cardio exercise, think of all the side benefits to biking instead of driving:

1. Biking is good for the environment

    Unlike driving, biking allows you to lower your carbon footprint. You don't need to use gas and you don't have to worry about vehicle emissions. You will be doing your part to fight air pollution, water pollution and sound pollution.

2. Less traffic

    Just think of all that time you can get stuck in traffic on the road. With biking, you can avoid a great deal of traffic. Soaring past cars that are waiting at lights will most likely allow your spirits to soar too!

3. Cost savings

    Many bikers have realized that biking has saved them a lot of cash. There are so many costs associated with using a car that we often don't even think about. For example, washing your car, parking your car, oil checks, insurance, gas, and tire replacements, etc. With a bike you can simply skip all of these costs. Think of the fun things you could do with that money!

4.   Meet new people

Often when you are on wheels, it gives you a chance to talk to and meet new people that you never would have before. You will start recognizing the other bike riders in your neighborhood and waving at them. If you decide to bike to work, you will start to recognize other bike commuters who pass through a similar part of town at the same time each day. Being able to give a nod or smile to others can do a lot to make you feel as though you are part of a friendly community.

Focus on What you Want

Everyone knows that exercise helps us drop weight when we are dieting. However, as it so happens, exercise also contributes many beneficial things to our lives. When it comes to thinking and feeling positive, allow yourself to shift your focus beyond just the exercise. After all, just thinking, "I should exercise because I am trying to lose weight" isn't really a powerful enough motivator to get us to truly get exercise to work on our behalf.

As ironic as it sounds, the word "exercise" fills many people with dread. They hear the word exercise, and the next thing that comes to their mind is "I don't want to..." or a sudden feeling of fatigue. However, when you can get your mind off the exercise itself and on to the bigger picture, you will have more success and better results.

Here are some factors to consider when you need an exciting reason to get out there and start exercising:

- **Cardiovascular exercises are good for our brains**

   Cardio exercise has been shown to keep our brains younger and healthier. This means that activity could actually help you think more effective. It is key for people who are more interested in intellectual pursuits than physical activity, to realize that the two are interconnected.

- **Exercise can cut food cravings**

   Do you want to kill two birds with one stone? Exercise also has the side benefit of curbing cravings. If you are feeling like eating, try going for a quick walk. Once your walk is over, see if you still feel like eating as much as you did at the start.

Just like the list that we came up for biking above, you can create similar lists for all types of activities and forms of exercise. Many have side benefits that can enhance your life and well-being in a variety of directions. Life is meant for exploring and trying new things. Go ahead and choose a new activity of exercise that you want to try, and start creating your own lists of side-benefits. It is time to focus beyond just the exercise in and of itself. Consider the many areas of your life that you will be improving.

Pace Yourself

Medicine has shown that even a brief amount of exercise is better for your body than being sedentary. Even a very short walk or lifting weights, which are light, can be of tremendous benefit. Although often people hear the term working out and envision themselves "killing themselves" and returning from the gym dripping with sweat, going to this level is really not necessary. In fact, working out *too* hard can sometimes actually not be as good for you as one would think.

The old motto "no pain, no gain" is detrimental to many people's outlook about exercise. It makes them feel as though if they agree to exercise, there will be lots of suffering involved. When your goal is lifelong fitness, more intensive workouts are usually not better.

Also keep in mind that when you are at the beginning of your days of working out, you should not push yourself as hard as one would push a seasoned athlete. You need to start off slowly and then gradually increase the intensity. If you push yourself too hard at first, you will actually get exhausted and likely need to take time off.

Many people hate exercise so much that when they are formulating their desires with the Law of Attraction they say something to the extent of, "I want to lose weight, but I don't have to have to do any exercise." This is one of those instances of thinking you want something, but in actuality if you got your wish you wouldn't want it at all. Be careful what you wish for! The fact of the matter is that science has shown that in order to be healthy, we need exercise. Yes, you could lose weight without exercising, but that would not be what was best for you and your body.

If you work out too intensely, it can actually prevent fat burning. In fact, overtaxing yourself with stressful exercise it can lead to cortisol production which can lead to fat getting stored in the lower abdomen. In fact, the higher the cortisol levels, the more likely that fat will get stored. This is one of the reasons why people who push themselves too hard working out get counterproductive results.

Overtraining can cause symptoms including:

- Pain and aches
- Fatigue and exhaustion
- Headaches

- Feeling unmotivated
- Illness
- Frequent Colds
- Injury

Vision Boards and Exercise

Remember the vision board about the best foods that we created in the food choices chapter? Now is the time to make a similar board about exercise. Just like with the food choice board, go ahead and get a board and place images of the words, and images that will be inspiring you to exercise. Again, this should be very personal for you.

The images can be of someone hiking to the top of a gorgeous mountain, skiers enjoying a fun winters day or even someone competing in a triathlon. Maybe what will inspire you to exercise is seeing images of yourself or other people in yoga positions. Perhaps you want to include images of washboard stomachs and trim legs. Again this really should be anything that gets you pumped up and motivated to exercise.

Now where the food choice vision board is on your refrigerator, place this exercise vision board somewhere that you can see it quite frequently. An ideal place would be the nightstand by your bed. When you wake up in the morning, take a look at all of these inspiring images and words in your vision board. Once you have been looking at this board every morning, the themes will start to seep into your subconscious and they will be with you all day long.

One of the reasons that vision boards work so well and we have stressed them throughout this book is that humans are very much visually oriented. In fact, a large portion of our brain is dedicated solely to sight! That is part of why our visualization works so well to bring forth our desires. So start the day off right by visualizing some details about your exercise in the day ahead.

Even if you don't exercise that particular day, the motivational images will build up to eventually create new agenda for your body, mind and spirit. If you don't think that you will have time to exercise that particular day, you certainly have the time to spend a few minutes looking at your vision board. You may even want to put your exercise vision board on the front door so you see it every time you leave the house!

Focus on What You Do Not Want

When it comes to getting motivated with exercise, one thing that works quite effectively is focusing on what you do not want. Lack of exercise, of course, can lead to a variety of diseases including diabetes, heart disease, stroke, high blood pressure and even cancer.

Exercise also has been shown to lower cortisol levels. Cortisol is in the body's circulatory system and is designed to protect us in times of stress. It is meant to be a short-term method of assisting us. Cortisol can be bad for you once it surpasses a certain level in the body. Cortisol promotes fat to be stored in the abdominal area. The reason the body does this is so that it will be easily accessible in case the "fight or flight response" is needed.

Cortisol levels can be controlled through exercise. In fact, some supplements like Relacore inhibit cortisol levels and that is how they claim to help people lose weight. Relaxation techniques help fight the amount of cortisol our body produces. So does some exercise like walking, breathing, yoga and Tai chi. Once our levels of stress come down, less cortisol is produced.

If not controlled, cortisol levels can lead not only to increased abdominal fat, but also cravings for sugar, blood sugar issues, thyroid problems, decreased bone density, high blood pressure, frequent illness, among other problems.

What has been shown to be the most effective in lowering cortisol levels is aerobic exercise. Cardio helps with stress management and it also removes cortisol from our systems. It helps release the by-products of cortisol.

Make Exercise Fun Again

When you were a kid you probably exercised all the time. Only you didn't think of it as exercise at the time. You might have played various sports, such as soccer or basketball. Soccer and basketball are two great examples of intense cardiovascular workouts that don't seem to be such when you are playing the game. Both sports involve running back and forth across a field or a court. The end result of this process is some of the best-conditioned athletes in the entire world.

Fun Activities and Sports To Keep You Motivated

1. Play basketball. Now this does not mean that you must join a basketball league and live, eat and breathe basketball. Just shooting some baskets and running around the court by you or with a friend can really work up a sweat.

2. Go bike riding. Riding a bike is obviously good exercise. If possible, pick a spot where you can get plenty of fresh air. After awhile, your body will become addicted to all that fresh air. You will feel so much better on a day-to-day basis that you will be motivated to go bike riding all the time.

3. Fresh air can be a powerful motivator. If you live in an area where you can safely go hiking, then by all means go for it! Getting out in nature is a super way to clear your head, get some exercise and give your lungs a break from all the pollution of the big city or congested suburbs.

4. If you played a sport as a kid or in high school or college, consider revisiting it. Of course, don't overdo it. If it has been years since you've hit a baseball, for example, don't spend three hours in the batting cages. Push that hard and the next morning you could be wondering why your back "doesn't work."

5. Consider physical activities that you haven't tried before. A great many people really enjoy activities such as bowling, cross-country skiing and swimming, for example. Take a look at the various sports and physical activities that you can do in your area and see which ones appeal to you.

6. Don't discount an activity as simple as a game of Frisbee with a friend. The bottom line is that you're running and burning off calories.

7. Find fun physical fitness in the mundane and ordinary. Simple acts can often be fun; especially if you are doing them with someone you like or love. Building a snowman or snow-woman is a great example of this principle in action. Lifting all of that snow can certainly burn some serious calories.

8. Video games. Yes video games can be a fun way of working out. Some very bright people realized that video games could be used to get people more active. Consider playing video games with interactive control schemes designed to get you off the couch. The Nintendo Wii is a great example of a video game that can burn some calories.

9. Do you have a dog? Going for a brisk walk or job with your four-legged buddy can be a healthy workout.

10. Dancing is an easy way to get active. This doesn't mean you have to put your earplugs in and head to the local pickup joint. You can stay and home and dance in the privacy of your own home. The key factor is to find activities that are fun.

The real point here is that you can stay motivated by keeping your physical activity fun. Of course you will be more likely to engage in physical activity if you are having a good time!

Often people let the word exercise conjure up negative emotions, before they even give thought and consideration to what they may actually enjoy doing. Frank has an interesting page on his website where he writes about interesting news stories on the topic of exercise. Many of these topics are so motivating, that they can practically get someone to overcome their fear and resistance to exercise. For example, one recent study by researchers at The University of Exeter showed that for people who are trying to quit smoking, just 15 minutes of exercise reduced people's tendency to smoke. This means that if you happen to be also trying to quit smoking, there is yet another impetus to get out there and start exercising.

Chapter 8
CONTINUING YOUR WEIGHT LOSS

"Not to have control over the senses is like sailing in a rudderless ship, bound to break to pieces on coming in contact with the very first rock." —*Gandhi*

Your new fit healthy body must be maintained with new habits and new ways of thinking. If you bounce back to old thought patterns, before you know it, the weight may have returned. In order to keep slim and trim, you must constantly maintain and monitor your thinking. The more that you cultivate new thoughts and behavioral patterns, however, the easier this process will be. Paying attention to the details of your food choices and diet are among the factors that will help you keep the weight off long term.

One of the great things about the Law of Attraction is that if you achieve a healthy weight by following its principles, you will be far less likely to be one of the statistics of people who lost weight only to gain it right back just a few weeks later. Remember, even the way that you frame your goal can manifest the result. As we discussed earlier in this book, if you have the goal of "losing weight" you will seek to find it again. And perhaps you will… just a few weeks later.

Many people simply fall back into their old patterns once they are off their diet. In fact, often we even eat more to make up for the weeks of denying oneself. This sets up a yo-yo situation. Through Law of Attraction, you can continue to monitor your thoughts and stay consistent to your goals. This means that you won't gain the weight back!

Consistency

One of the things that can keep the weight off is for you to remain consistent in your diet. This means that you will establish a pattern for the types of foods that you eat, and than only diverge from it once and again. This doesn't mean that you can't experiment and try new foods. It just means that you have pinned down your staples that benefit your body and your health. You also have set up consistent routines, getting certain fruits and veggies into your diet, exercise and drinking lots of water.

Most people who keep the weight off, also never leave themselves feeling hungry or deprived of food. The Mayo Clinic's Health Letter issued a report about a study of 5000 people who had lost weight and kept of the weight. Most of these people lost at least 72 pounds and everyone had kept at least 30 pounds off for good. Since 1994, the National Weight Control Registry has also been tracking people who lost weight and kept it off.

So what do these people do to keep the weight off?

- **They eat a low fat, low calorie diet.**
- **They get physical activity.**

   Almost all of the people in this study exercised regularly. Of the forms of exercise, walking turned out to be the most common. The common amount of exercise for people in this study was about an hour a day.

- **They eat breakfast every day.**

   This point is another one supporting the theory that you should never under eat to the point where you feel deprived. Eating breakfast everyday sets you up to have energy and fuel throughout the day. Of course, you want to carefully select what you eat for breakfast. (10 pancakes with syrup every day are not going to be beneficial towards keeping off the weight!)

- **They monitor their weight every day.**

   Although stepping on the scale every day may sound unpleasant to you, it turns out that this is major factor among people who have lost weight and kept it off. These people were likely to weigh themselves every day. This routine helps them become mindful of when they might be going "off the wagon" and need to readjust.

Another reason that weighing yourself every day is important is that it will give you a clear ability to reward yourself and visually see your results. You can look at the scale and see you are at the weight that you once only dreamed of being. You have manifested your reality. When you step on the scale every day and see that you are still at your desired weight, you can pat yourself on the back and feel proud of yourself.

The longer that you can keep the weight off, the more likely that your new body will be permanent. For the people in this study, if they kept their weight off for 2 years, they were 50% less likely to gain back the weight.

Your Old Patterns

If you realize that you may be slipping back into your old patterns, this is a real warning sign that you may start gaining back the weight. Now, this doesn't mean that when you are at the weight you want, you can't reward yourself with a cookie or cake every now and then. There is a difference between an occasional treat and slipping into a pattern of binge eating.

Remember that if you go ahead and start eating more sugar, your body is going to start craving the sugar again. It is no coincidence. Sugar is indeed addictive. This means that when you do indulge, you just need to monitor yourself and watch for the effects of the food you ate to potentially pop up and try to control you.

At any time, you can revert back to the six steps of *You Can Attract It*. Go back and remember the second and third steps—What You Don't Want and What You Want. Reconnect with the Law of Attraction whenever you feel yourself slipping. Acknowledge how much the Law of Attraction has already assisted you towards your goals. Connecting with what you want is always a good method for establishing new healthy habits and letting go of old ones.

Your Old Patterns and Your Old Friends

Dropping those extra pounds is a journey that you might have to do without certain friends or others that you currently associate with frequently. Many people will not share your desire to get healthy and stay that way. If this is the case then you might have to reduce your exposure to those people. Negative energy is counterproductive. If your friends, family or others are sending it in your direction, the bottom line is that you need to protect yourself in order to protect your goals.

Negative influences that threaten to impede your progress must be taken seriously. This doesn't mean that you scream, "You are negative energy man! Get away from me with all your negative energy stuff!" It simply means that you have to take into consideration the people around you and how they may be influencing your decisions and actions.

Obviously, if you have a friend that is scornful or resentful of your attempts to drop a few pounds, you might have no real alternative but to avoid that friend. Achieving your fitness goals may mean prioritizing those goals above friendships and other associations. While this is easy to state, it might be difficult to put into action. For this reason, it may be necessary to make a serious and dedicated resolution to clear your life of negativity. Remember your true goal is to drop pounds and get healthy.

The Benefits of Drinking Water

Our bodies are mostly made of water—between 55% and 75% in fact! Many people spend each day not feeling well simply because they are not getting enough water. In order to keep our bodies functioning optimally, we must drink water. Every day our breathing alone expels 2-4 cups of water from the body. Water also leaves our body through sweating and urination.

> Many people spend each day not feeling well simply because they are not getting enough water.

Think about all the water that we lose. Doesn't it make sense to rehydrate with water? Often people with problems with weight make the mistake of drinking soda instead of water. This is a big mistake, as not only does soda not hydrate our bodies, it fills us full of toxins that we do not need. There are a wide variety of important reasons to drink water, especially when you are maintaining your weight and health. If you are exercising, for example, you are going to need extra water to make up for the water lost during exercise.

Here are some common symptoms that come from lack of water other than thirst, which is of course on the list.

- Fatigue
- Headaches or Migraines
- Weakness
- Lightheadedness and inability to focus
- Muscle weakness or cramps
- Less urine
- Dry Skin
- Kidney problems
- Blood pressure problems

Most doctors recommend eight 8-ounce glasses of water a day. This is just an estimate for how much you need, as this number changes a bit based on your size, sex, and other specifics. All of the critical functions of the body are dependant on drinking enough water. If you are trying to reach your ideal body weight or keep your ideal body weight, you need to continuously flush the body's waste products out. Water also carries nutrients from our food through our body. It transports the nutrients into our cells.

Also drinking water can reduce hunger pangs. Often when we think that we are hungry, we really just need water. If you are feeling hungry, before eating some food, simply try drinking some water and see how you feel afterwards.

Water also supports the goal of radiant health. After all, think of how a plant looks when it doesn't get enough water. Like a plant, we can also begin to look dry, dull and shriveled when we don't get enough water. Water is great for our skin and keeps it looking soft and wrinkle free. It also helps replenish skin and maintain skin elasticity. Water also can improve the appearance of our hair and nails. When you think of all the amazing things water can do for your health, you really have to wonder why anyone would choose something like soda instead of a glass of water. The more you understand the necessity of water to your body, the more frequently you will choose it over other drinks.

When you are drinking more water, you will also feel more energized and ready to exercise. Your muscles will feel stronger and more ready for physical activity. Also you will have fewer incidences of muscle cramps during the exercise periods. Because you will feel so much better when you are drinking enough water, it will keep you in a good mood and ready to keep achieving your goals with the Law of Attraction.

Purify Your Water

Eating healthy foods is a often given a good deal of attention and focus in books and articles about health. However, what is often overlooked, but is very important is healthy water. In recent years, the nation's water supply has become increasingly polluted with a variety of chemicals and harmful compounds. Unfortunately this is not a myth. A good step toward better health isn't just drinking more water, but taking steps towards drinking healthier, cleaner water.

With this issue of water in mind it is a good idea to invest in some system for purifying your drinking water. There are a great many ways of doing this and while it might take some research its definitely worth the time. One of the easiest steps is to simply buy a water pitcher filtering system. These water pitcher filtering systems are available in most stores are relatively inexpensive and have been proven to work. While the most definitely do not remove all pollutants from water, they are certainly better than nothing at all!

Eating Small Meals

When you are seeking to end struggles with your weight for good, another suggestion is to eat small frequent meals throughout the day as opposed to large meals. Many people call eating small meals throughout the day "grazing." This can mean eating every 3-4 hours. Yes, we were always taught to eat 3 square meals a day, but as it turns out, this system is less effective for keeping a healthy weight and feeling one's best. Part of the problem with the 3 meals a day philosophy is that it encourages a massive dinner when you get home from work. Even worse, a big dessert could follow this massive dinner!

People who have trouble with their weight often skip meals and then sit down and eat feast. Skipping meals can put stress on your body. It can also put you in a bad mood. It is also not ideal for your metabolism to eat a bunch of food in one sitting and then go for many hours without eating. When you aren't feeling at your best, you are less likely to be manifesting your ideal vision via the Law of Attraction.

There is a big difference between grazing and snacking. Snacking is when you eat food to keep yourself at bay all day, but it is things like candy, cookies and other unhealthy snacks. So what should you eat in each meal when you graze? Try to keep it so each meal has fresh fruits and vegetables, proteins and healthy fats or grains. This way you are getting the nutrition that you need, but again, you are spreading this nutrition throughout the day.

Also when you are skipping meals it is not a reaffirming statement to yourself. Instead, you are telling yourself, in essence, that dropping pounds is difficult and takes a degree of suffering. As we have discussed in this book, this is not the best message to be sending your body. You also do not want to send the universe this message. Instead, you want to send the message that you consistently fuel your body throughout the day with nutritious food.

As we all know, there is another big problem with eating big meals. Think about Thanksgiving. Even though what you eat may be delicious, you typically get drowsy afterwards and maybe even feel as though you need a nap. When you eat small meals throughout the day, you will be less likely to have these swings in energy levels. When you eat multiple meals throughout the day, you are also telling your body that it never needs to be hungry. Your body will get out of the pattern of every having cravings. Also your calories will be spread throughout the day. Eating small meals really is a formula for looking and feeling your best.

Eating Small Meals—It's Important For Your Health

Eating small meals is very important as it puts less strain on your heart and other vital organs. Science and medicine know that eating large meals can put serious strain on the body. By choosing to eat smaller meals, you are making a very important decision in improving your overall health.

Smaller meals also mean less serious meal choice mistakes. If you are in the habit of eating smaller meals and you "fall off the diet wagon," at least your transgression was a small meal transgression and not a big meal transgression. Smaller meals are smarter meals for a large variety of reasons. Also with smaller meals you have a much clearer idea of what kind of food you are putting into your body and how that food makes you feel.

As we saw in the above study of people who have lost weight and kept it off, all of these people eat breakfast. Another important thing about breakfast is that it jump-starts your metabolism. When you eat throughout the day, you keep your metabolism running efficiently. Of course, when you have a lower metabolism it is more difficult to lose weight. What we want ideally is for our metabolism to be running effectively and burning fat and calories throughout the day.

Another problem with skipping a meal is that when you finally do get some food, you are more likely to overeat. Skipping meals can also cause our blood sugar levels to drop. Again, this can lead to binging or overeating at the next meal. When you are eating every couple of hours, you really can only eat so much food before you get full. You will find that you no longer even want to overeat. You just lose interest in the prospect of gorging yourself.

Keep Reading About Beneficial Foods and Exercise

Another tip that is instrumental for keeping the weight off is to become a lifelong learner about all things that are healthy for your body. If you make learning about health and nutrition a priority, than the results will continue to manifest as a result of your thinking and feelings. You will consistently be thinking about nutrition and what is the best thing to do and eat to benefit your body.

There are a number of top notch website, newsletters and publications that will keep you informed on all advancements and studies that are related to health, nutrition, and weight. As we have mentioned, Frank has a fantastic website with a variety of health and nutrition related resources. He also has a page that he updates with new stories from the science and medical community about exercise and nutrition. His twitter and Facebook pages also seek to inform people about this type of news. It is a good idea to visit Frank's site and also keep your eye on similar resources.

Another good idea is to visit message boards and forums that are frequented by people who have also kept the weight off. If you can find a community where people also achieved great results in their life through the Law of Attraction that is also ideal. Just logging into a community every day or every few days and reading inspiring stories and tips from likeminded people can do wonders to keep you on target. People will also post suggestions for exercises, beneficial habits, and new low calorie recipes that you can try.

Sometimes when you are working on your health and dropping pounds, you can begin to feel very isolated. We are humans and we need community. Being able to connect with other people who are going through similar types of experiences can be enormously beneficial.

However, here is one word of caution. Try not to fall for any fad diets that may derail you. Once you have achieved your weight that you are seeking, you have done it! Keep your confidence level high. You did it yourself, you do not need any of the diet products, services or gimmicks that you see promoted around you. There will always be marketers who are trying to make a quick buck off of people who are desperate. You certainly don't want to get lumped into this crowd of people who could potentially bring you down.

If you try something new even if it sounds good at first, it will likely derail your progress. For example, there are diets that say you can eat whatever you want and lose weight promising to be the "magic bullet." For example, there is the cookie diet, various weight loss supplements and pills, and cleanses. Just remember that the real magic bullet is the Law of Attraction and your positive thinking and actions.

Forgive Yourself

Another important item to stress when it comes to keeping weight off for a lifetime is to not be so hard on yourself. Eventually, you are going to have a day where you eat things that you know are wrong and bad for you. It could be a moment of weakness, a social gathering, or a stressful occasion. There are a number of moments throughout life that cause even the best healthiest eater in the world to cave in to some treat or another.

> ... when it comes to keeping weight off for a lifetime is to not be so hard on yourself.

When and if this happens, just remember to not be so tough on yourself. If you have been eating healthy foods and have been on a healthy routine, a day or two of "bad" eating won't amount to anything. Sometimes people who have lost weight find that when they lose weight and then have a day where they screw up it sends them into a deep despair. All of a sudden, all of those old feelings about weight loss being hard and about failure resurface. Before they know it these thoughts and feelings can snowball into more overeating. Then before you know it they may be back in the same old patterns once again.

If you have a day where you failed at what you ate, forget about the temporary situation. Think about the big picture. You have already come so far. You have already made real changes towards your new healthy body. If you are patient and keep what you do want in mind, your misstep will have absolutely no impact towards your current and future level of success. Certainly, don't get depressed and disheartened about your failure. Everyone experiences setbacks. Often set backs are a learning experience we need to get to the next level of success.

Part Two

HEALTHY LIVING AND EATING

Chapter 9

THE LAW OF ATTRACTION AND LIFESTYLE CHOICES

"Eating a vegetarian diet, walking everyday, and meditating is considered radical. Allowing someone to slice your chest open and graft your leg veins in your heart is considered normal and conservative." —Dr. Dean Ornish

There can be little doubt that our lifestyle choices can profoundly impact our lives in almost every conceivable way. The results of our lifestyle choices are rarely more evident than in our health. The health consequences of poor health choices can radiate out in directions that are both obvious as well as more obtuse.

The fact that poor health choices can lead to dire health consequences has been well promoted by the media and society at large. For example, most of us know that if we smoke packs of cigarettes a day for years. we are dramatically increasing our risk of developing lung cancer and other cancers.

Another prime example of lifestyle choices impacting our health is in the realm of alcohol consumption. Like smoking or using tobacco products, alcohol can have negative health consequences. Most people know that consuming too much alcohol can lead to severe organ damage. Those who abuse alcohol can face liver disease and problems with their kidneys and that is just for starters.

The Difference Between Alcohol, Tobacco and Food Choices

The fact that alcohol and tobacco products are bad for you is widely known and recognized by most in society. In fact, you may be rolling your eyes reading this chapter so far. You might be thinking, "Of course, I know all this…" However, consider this point for a moment. Once upon a time and not too long ago, smoking cigarettes and drinking was promoted in the mainstream media as healthy and perfectly acceptable. Obviously, that would seem ridiculous today. But it is interesting to note how the mainstream opinion of what is and what isn't healthy can change dramatically. It has only been in the last few years that people have begun to take a close and careful look at diet's impact on health. Yet, there is increasing awareness that our dietary choices can quite literally end in premature death.

Even though the media has begun to give a considerable more attention to diet and health, there is still a tremendous amount of confusion regarding the topic. In a sense this is understandable. The message that smoking and alcohol carry a risk with them is easy enough to understand. The fact that both products carry a health risk with them was a pretty straightforward message. Those who asked the question, "What kind of alcohol is bad for me?" got a simple answer. "All kinds of alcohol are bad for you."

Sadly, where food and its impact on health are concerned, the problem is infinitely more complex. Some foods are good, some foods are bad and some foods are somewhere in between. There isn't a tobacco product that is "somewhere in between" as they are all pretty much bad for you. The complexity of the diet and food is thus much more complex. Thus, people can be excused for being confused especially when seemingly reputable sources dole out conflicting and confusing information.

Stopping To Think About Your Health and Food Choices

A key move for anyone who is looking to lose weight is to begin questioning his or her own perceptions and ideas regarding food and diet. You should stop and ponder what ideas are shaping your thinking. Here are a few questions that you should ask yourself regarding diet, food and your thoughts on the topic.

How Do You See And Think About Food?

1. Where do you get most of your food information?

2. Who do you see as being the most notable and respected sources of information?

3. What do you think is the most reputable source for information on health and nutrition?

4. How often have you asked a health care professional about nutrition and health?

5. Before reading this book, how many books had you read about health and nutrition in the last year?

6. How many articles have your head on health and nutrition in the last year?

7. How often do you visit health and nutrition websites or blogs in a given year?

8. When was the last time you took a class that had a health and nutrition component?

9. What impute do you receive from your friends and family about food and nutrition?

10. How much of your socializing involves food?

11. When is the last time you've learned a health or nutrition fact that changed your mind about health and nutrition?

12. When is the last time that you had a health fact or nutrition fact change the way you ate?

13. Before reading this book, how confident were you that you could learn new information that would impact your diet and health?

It is important that you answer the above questions openly and honestly with yourself. You should pause to contemplate the answers. As you may already suspect where, how and who you are getting your information regarding health and nutrition from is, in all likelihood, greatly impacting your health choices. For this reason it is quite important that you carefully think through how you are reaching your conclusions about health and nutrition and equally importantly where you are getting this information from on a regular basis.

Like Attracts Like

More than likely the core Law of Attraction concept that "like attracts like" is now firmly fixed in your mind. Just as the Law of Attraction works to help people make more money, the exact same thing holds true for being healthy and dropping weight. For example, if you were surrounding yourself with people who were negative about the possibility of making money, you would have to distance yourself from them. This is due to the fact that you would benefit from shielding yourself from their negativity. In order to successfully move towards making money, you would want to associate yourself with positive thoughts and actions surrounding your income.

Now let's take a look at getting to your healthy weight for a moment. If you find that you are surrounding yourself with people who have horrible health habits, then it may be necessary to take drastic actions. You simply cannot associate with people who have horrible health habits and who are negative about your health related goals.

Even if you are incredibly strong willed, their thoughts and vibrational energy can still impact your life.

Evaluating Your Associations

If your health goal is to shed some pounds, then you definitely don't want someone around that is constantly telling you that dropping those pounds is next to impossible. Wouldn't it seem like nonsense to spend a great deal of time with someone that was telling you that your goals and plans were extremely hard? In what possible context could such behavior make any sense? The fact of the matter is that you should be associating only with those who support your thoughts that losing weight is easy.

The Law of Attraction will always be guiding and controlling your life. Therefore, you must be very careful about who you associate with. As it turns out one of the major lifestyle changes that you may need to make is to reconsider who you choose to associate with and why. Many of the questions you were asked to ponder earlier in this chapter directly correlate to this point. You need to evaluate whom you are associating with and what kind of information on health and nutrition you are receiving from them.

The bottom line is that you shouldn't make your job of dropping the pounds any more difficult than it might naturally already be. Part of using the Law of Attraction in relation to your lifestyle choices is to recognize that your associations may be playing a major role in your ability to succeed.

Evaluating Your Friends, Family And Associates

For some perplexing reason it is considered almost taboo to evaluate whether or not you should be associating with your family and to a lesser extent your friends, but the facts are that you should be. Anyone who is looking to accomplish a goal, whether it is to make money, get in shape or drop some pounds, needs to contemplate whom they are spending their time with and how those people are impacting them.

Your goal is to associate with people that will help you achieve you goals by being positive and providing you with moral support or concrete suggestions. If you have family members who are being negative about your health and nutrition goals, it might be necessary to start spending less time with them. Of course, the first approach is to tell them your concerns and see if this leads to behavior modification. Ultimately, however, it might be necessary to ask yourself, "How badly do I want to reach my goals?"

Remember that you make the choice to spend time with the people around you. You might not be able to get away from the guy in the desk next to you, but odds are you can reduce your exposure to other negative people in your life. Here are a few questions that you should be asking concerning your associations.

1.   What are my family's attitude towards health and nutrition?

2.   What is the attitude of my friends towards nutrition and health?

3.   Are my friends and family generally in good health?

4.   How do my friends and family react when I tell them I want to get in shape?

5.   How do my friends and family react when I tell them I want to drop some pounds?

6.   Have any friends or family made fun of you for your health goals? How would you generally rate their level of support?

7.   Do your friends and family offer to give you help to reach your health and weight goals?

8.   Once your friend and family knew about your goal to drop weight or get in shape did their behavior change? If so, how?

9.   When you are spending time with your friends and family do they respect your dietary choices?

10. Do your friends and family put you in situations where you are likely to go off your diet? Do they present you with your favorite foods or encourage you to "just have a bite or two?"

As you ask yourself these questions, you need to remember that you are the one that is living with the health consequences of your lifestyle choices and not them. If you are surrounding yourself with negative people, you are effectively making a lifestyle choice right there on the spot.

How To Make Better Choices

A sense of loyalty often drives people to continue to associate with friends and family, but this is a lifestyle choice and luxury that the Law of Attraction simply does not afford us. If you are striving to drop pounds, then you will have to carefully think through your decisions regarding your associations.

Lets say you have a friend from high school that you talk to every few weeks, however, this friend is overweight and thinks that getting healthier is a waste of time. Just because you are in a pattern where you constantly speak to her doesn't mean you have to continue doing so. Now may be the time that you have to cut off (at least temporarily) some of your contacts.

Clearly, the power to associate with those with whom you are comfortable is natural. Falling back into that pattern is clearly easy. With this in mind, it is necessary that you develop and embrace strategies that will help you find ways to avoid those who might be negatively impacting your health choices. Again it should be reiterated that your associations are lifestyle choices that can greatly influence your other lifestyle choices, such as what foods you eat.

Strategies For Making Better Association Choices

1. Try and associate with those who support your health goals.

2. Discuss your new health goals and your desire to drop weight with your friends and family. It may be very important to underscore how important reaching these goals are for you. If you are persistent in how important these goals are for you, you may very well get good results. You may inspire your friends and family to start following your lead and become healthier themselves.

3. Take practical steps to minimize the opportunity for friends and family to impact your activities. If, for example, you know that your friends are going to your favorite restaurant that serves fattening, unhealthy food, don't go along with them. Instead tell them that you can meet them somewhere else afterwards.

4. Explore new activities. By doing so you may make new friends who are more in line with your health goals.

5. Explore joining organizations and clubs where you are more likely to meet people who are likely to be more in line with your health goals. This could be a raw food group, a hiking group or a healthy cooking class.

6. Consider working with a nutritionist for both practical advice and for a sounding board regarding your health goals. In this fashion, a nutritionist can serve as a partial support network for goals, such as your goal to drop weight.

7. Just as a nutritionist may help serve as a partial support network for your health goals, the same can be stated for a personal trainer. Just remember that not all personal trainers are equally qualified or motivated. You should do your research and don't be afraid to switch to another personal trainer.

8. If possible see if you can find a "healthy eating buddy" that can help you with your dieting goals. In this way, you will have someone in your corner who can help you meet your health goals.

9. Having a "healthy eating buddy" is very important and can help in a variety of ways, ranging from moral support to actual companionship. This buddy can even help you find new ways to meet your diet and health goals.

Remember To Be Proactive

Much of the trick concerning negative associations is to remain proactive. You need to be constantly reviewing and thinking about your associations and how they are impacting your lifestyle choices. Imagine for a moment that a bunch of work friends are going out after work for a drinking and eating marathon. While you might want to go, you know that your diet will suffer greatly. You may very well be tempted, but you should refrain from going. You must keep your focus on your goals of optimum health.

Instead find something else to do. This underscores the value of, if necessary, developing new hobbies, interest and friends. If you have new friends, for example, and you are in a particularly social mood simply call up some of your new friends.

Important Lifestyle Choices That You Must Make

Developing and cultivating a climate in which you are more likely to achieve your health goals is the most important lifestyle choice that you can make. There are, however, other critical steps that must be taken if you are serious about dropping pounds and increasing your overall level of physical fitness. While some of these lifestyle choices may not be easy, they are quite necessary. Failing to adopt these choices will have potentially serious long-term consequences for both your health and your goals. Phrased another way, these lifestyle choices are a big deal.

No More Sugar

You might be rubbing your eyes in disbelief, but you have indeed read this correctly. Ultimately, the less sugar you consume, the better off you will be. Sugar is simply not good for your body as it produces a variety of negative health consequences. Alco consider for just a moment that sugar has no nutritional value.

When you consume sugar, you are effectively wasting your calories. That is something that someone intent on dropping pounds can simply not do, especially on a regular basis. With this in mind, you will have to find ways to eliminate sugar from your diet. There are alternatives and strategies that you can use to consume less and less sugar. Here are a few ideas that you should find very useful.

Tips And Ideas For Reducing Sugar Consumption

1. Don't try to quite "cold turkey." If you have been consuming a good deal of sugar for most of your life (such as two or three spoons in your coffee every day), then you are somewhat dependent on the stuff. Attempting to quit all sugar instantly might literally drive you mad. Slowly decrease the amount of sugar you are using over weeks so that your body doesn't crash.

2. Explore healthier alternatives to sugar. Honey is a great alternative to sugar and while it most definitely contains sugar, there are several important differences between sugar and honey. Organic honey and organic raw honey are not processed like sugar. Secondly, honey has numerous health benefits such as anti-bacterial properties. Try switching to honey as a sweetener. Odds are that this switch will not be as difficult as you think. Agave is made from cactus and it is another great alternative to sugar.

3. Molasses is another wonderful sweetening alternative, but it doesn't work in everything due to its taste. So you will have to experiment to see where you can use molasses and in what foods you like it. Molasses, especially if you shop around for a high-quality brand, can contain a surprising amount of nutrition for the calories. High-quality molasses is high in iron, magnesium, B Vitamins and calcium. You simply will not receive that from sugar. Buy organic molasses whenever possible as well.

4. You may have not heard of Xylitol, but many find it to work great as a sweetener. Made from the bark of a tree, Xylitol doesn't act like sugar in the body and actually has health benefits as well. Xylitol has been used extensively in Finland for decades. Numerous studies have shown that it is safe for consumption. In terms of health benefits, Xylitol appears to have the ability to inhibit tooth decay. So here you have a sweetener that can replace sugar most of the time that also has health benefits. Xylitol can have one side effect, however, so go slowly at first. Some have experienced lose stools with Xylitol, but this is the exception, not the rule.

5. Don't confuse reducing your sugar consumption with switching out a using some sort of chemical based artificial sweetener. In fact using artificial sweeteners is one of the worst things you can do for your body. Artificial sweeteners have been shown in numerous medical and scientific studies to cause diseases such as cancer in lab animals. Don't use artificial sweeteners. (In fact, you are probably better off with sugar!)

6. If you feel a sugar craving coming on, reach for a natural alternative. One great natural alternative to sugar is to snack on dried fruit. Dried fruit is high in natural sugars and may help you deal with your sweet tooth. Additionally, dried fruit is easily carried and will not spoil. This means that you can always have some handy as you can keep some in your car or at work.

7. Just as dried fruit help with your sugar cravings, so can food such as watermelon, grapes or pineapple, for example. All three of these fruits are almost like candy and have health benefits as well. Canned pineapples are a great pick, as they are available year round and will not spoil.

Reduce Your Salt Intake

You can live without processed sugar and artificial sweeteners, but the fact is that your body needs salt to survive. That stated, however, most people consume entirely too much salt. Consuming too much salt can lead to serious health consequences, thus, you need to take steps to reduce your salt intake whenever possible.

Ways To Reduce Your Salt Intake

1. Switching to Himalayan salt is one of the smartest moves you can make in regards to salt consumption. Himalayan salt is far purer than conventional salt and has trace minerals. Further a little Himalayan salt goes a long way, thus offsetting its higher cost. There is also the side benefit that it makes food taste much better, just try it!

2. Spices are good for you, so try reducing salt and adding other spices to your food. The result will be tastier food that is better for you.

3. Seek out and locate hidden sources of sodium. Manufacturers love to put salt in everything. It is evevn in foods that you wouldn't expect such as ice cream. This means that you really need to be looking at your labels quite intensely.

4. Learn to prepare a few healthy low-sodium meals and make them in advance. In the end your body will thank you.

Remember To Be Optimistic

Being upbeat and optimistic about dropping pounds and your health is a great step in the right direction. Remember what the Law of Attraction states—that you will get more of what you focus on. This is part of the reason that you need to concern yourself with who you associate with as well as where you receive your health and nutrition information

> ... you need to remain focused, positive, and willing to experiment and try new paths.

from on a daily basis. You can achieve your health goals, but you need to remain focused, positive, and willing to experiment and try new paths.

Chapter 10

THE POWER OF BEING ACTIVE

"Movement is the process of the Universe. So move.
Do something. Anything. But do not stand still. Do not remain
'on the horns of a dilemma.' Do not fence sit." —Neale Donald Walsch

Being active means that you are not inactive. Now while that sounds obvious, and it is, the real life implications are profound. If one is active then change is far, far more likely than being inactive. An inactive person is simply not getting as much done or attempting to do as much as an active person. There is just no way around this point; it's just a fact.

Active people change their lives and they often even change the world; whereas, inactive people do so with far less irregularity. The inactive person may have the vision, imagination and knowledge to accomplish something, but if he or she is not active, then there isn't too much chance of the dreams ever becoming reality.

The Law of Attraction can help dreams become reality via breathing life into what we envision, yet this is not to state that there is no work involved in the process. Sitting about envisioning that you will shed pounds only to eat the same food you've always eaten, in the same portion and not working out, will not yield results. The person that is going to shed the pounds is the person that is active in a variety of ways.

Shedding pounds and achieving your weight loss goals are about being active and dynamic. It is about making changes to your past life and embracing new possibilities and new ways of doing things. You simply can't not sit by passively and expect that your life will suddenly change for the better. In fact, if you sit around long enough your life most certainly will change. But who is to say you will have a hand in that change?

Being active means that you have a great say in your own destiny. Of course, this means that being inactive puts you in the passive position of waiting for events to impact upon you. For example, the result of physical inactivity will eventually be a decrease in overall health or even mental health.

Being Active Means You Can Achieve Your Goals

By all means you should want to be active. You should seek out a plan of action that will help you be effective and active. A plan of action will help you take the steps you need towards accomplishing your goals.

Think about it for a moment; in order to achieve your goal to shed pounds you will no doubt need to expend energy in some form. Even if you manage to drop the pounds strictly through diet, you still must expend the mental energy necessary to make the dietary changes that come along with a calorie reduction. You will need to pick out new foods, do research on new foods or perhaps consult a nutritionist. In a very basic and real way, change in the universe is a result of energy being expended.

Thus, you need two things in order to get your goal of shedding pounds into action. The first component that you will need is a plan. A well thought out plan of action is critical for anyone who wants to actively change his or her life. The second necessary component is energy. The mental and physical energy necessary to change your life is critical. For without that energy, the best plans in the world can be rendered useless.

The Benefits of Exercise and Achieving Your Goals

Exercise works to actually increase energy levels. As it turns out, exercising will not only make you feel better, but it gives you more energy as well. You may have heard of the "runner's high" that runners often report receiving from running. It turns out that this is based firmly in science. Runners do, in fact, quite literally get addicted to running, due to the fact that it feels good. Weight lifters and others who work out a great deal are also prone to experience the addictive effects of exercising.

So why does exercise make one feel so good? The human body is literally wired to make it want to be physically fit. When you exercise, especially with vigorous and more demanding exercises, your body releases endorphins. The endorphins are the body's feel good drug and this, of course, explains in part, why working out is prone to make you feel good and may even give you a "runner's high."

If you are working out your will feel better, not just physically, but mentally as well. You will quite literally have feel good chemicals running through your body. Of course, working out will also make you feel physically better as you are likely to have less aches and pains. Working out will strengthen your muscles and tendons making it less likely that you will become injured. This means that working out will make you feel better physically and mentally and in fact the two are intertwined and interconnected.

Feeling strong and physically fit will boost your confidence levels and also reduces the levels of the stress hormone cortisol in the body. You might remember from our previous chapter that cortisol is the dangerous stress hormone that can cause all sorts of serious problems ranging from infertility, to a weakening of your immune system, to literally causing you to age. Working out helps reduce the levels of cortisol in your body, and this can mean that you are less likely to feel and see the effects of aging. Further, it also means that you are less likely to get colds and flus. This means less time being sick, which is of course, great news.

Its All Interconnected

Have you picked up the pattern here yet? Once again, there is a mind and body connection between working out and mental health. Working out will help you cultivate a positive mental outlook, in part, via the endorphins that are released. Your life will also improve due to the fact that you feel better physically. This, in turn, makes you feel better mentally. It is indeed all rolled into one.

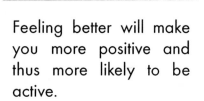

Feeling better will make you more positive and thus more likely to be active.

Feeling better will make you more positive and thus more likely to be active. If you are more physically active and you have more energy, you are more likely to go after your goals, whether it is shedding a few pounds or another goal. Additionally, you are more likely to set up and establish new goals. Without a surplus of energy you would not be striving toward your goals and you most certainly would not be sitting up new goals. You might be thinking, "Who knew exercising was so vital to achieving my goals?" Yet, as it turns out this is most definitely the case.

How Being More Active Will Change Your Life

- **Being Active Means New Horizons**

  While using the term "new horizons" might seem a bit clichéd, there is no doubt that the term is most definitely applicable. By doing everything you can to make yourself more active, you are opening up new horizons for yourself. With your new energy you will tackle new endeavors and experience new ways of living. Here are some additional points to consider when it comes to how physical activity can improve your life.

- **Being More Active Will Keep Your Mind Off Food**

  More energy could very well lead you towards being more socially active. You may find that you have the desire and determination to "get out there" and meet people. This may range from joining new organizations to simply reconnecting with old friends.

  As a byproduct, if you are out and active, you are likely not focused on food, your diet or eating. This increases the chances of dropping pounds and keeping them off. Once again, it all began with becoming more physically active.

- **Being More Active Will Help Your Friends and Family**

  Consider your friends and family for a moment. Often we forget that we touch all those around us. In our celebrity-obsessed culture, it is quite easy to forget that everyone has someone that they are impacting. More than likely there are scores and scores of people that you are impacting. Have you ever been motivated to shed a little weight after seeing a friend, relative or even an acquaintance do so? By exercising, dropping weight and getting in shape, you might very well serve as an example to your friends and family that they too can turn their health around.

- **Being More Active Could Mean A Better Job or Finding Love**

  Being more active means that you will be more fit. This could, in turn, mean that your confidence level will be boosted even higher. A more "socially active you" combined with a "more confident you" may lead to interesting opportunities no matter what you desire. If you are looking for a better or different kind of job and you expand your social spheres, in time you might meet someone that leads you to that new job. You might make business connections or find the love of your life as well.

- **Active People Get More "Breaks" In Life**

  Often it is thought that this person or that person is getting all the breaks, but the truth of the matter is that active people create more opportunities for themselves. By simply becoming more active you are creating a host of new opportunities for yourself. Imagine two men, Dave and Ken, are seeking a significant others and are having no luck. Dave doesn't do much beyond going to work and occasionally the store. However, Ken has a host of hobbies and is engaged in all sorts of other social activities. Ken is involved in numerous clubs ranging from a bowling league to a reading group to a kayaking club to name just a few.

The act of "getting out there" creates a host of new opportunities for Ken that Dave will never have. Consider this point; Ken doesn't even have to meet his significant other at any of these clubs. Perhaps he makes a friend who has a coworker that he or she feels is perfect for Ken.

It is an often forgotten fact that the vast majority of people, who form long-term relationships, met either at work or through friends. Having a mutual friend give the "stamp of approval" can go along way toward creating a friendlier dating environment. The bottom line is that, most of the time Ken will find a date long, long before Dave.

This is just another way that being active can greatly assist you in meeting your goals. Now if you switch out dating with finding a job or business partners the same holds true. The more connections you make the more opportunities for something good to happen there are.

By simply becoming more engaged with the world, the possibilities of all of these things happening skyrockets. Think of it this way, who is more likely to get what they want out of life, the person who is sitting in their home or apartment or the person who is "out there" working to meet other people and working to change their life? The answer is pretty clear.

Another Secret About Being More Active

There is another benefit to exercise that many people don't know about even though there has been a good deal of research and press on the topic. Exercise helps you sleep better. Have you ever noticed that it is easier to sleep when you have had a good workout or even a long walk? The lifestyle that most of us now live is not what the human body evolved to do. We were not meant to spend our days sitting in chairs in office talking to other people or staring at electronic boxes and typing away. Instead we were meant to be moving, climbing and even sprinting for short distances.

Thus the facts are that being more active can increase our physical health in ways that many people simply don't consider. The fact that sleep can help you sleep better is a very big point in favor of getting physically active. Research shows that sleep helps with wound healing and that a lack of sleep can actually hinder the immune system's ability to function properly. Of course, a lack of sleep most definitely will impact one's ability to be active. Sleepy people don't feel like doing too much, do they?

By getting quality sleep, you are making yourself feel better in ways both obvious and not so obvious. Quality sleep, and enough of it, means that you are rested enough that you feel like being active. It also means that you are helping your body stay healthy through boosting your immune system and helping wounds heal. Obviously if you are sick, then you probably won't feel much like being "Mr. or Mrs. Active."

If you are still not convinced that skipping sleep is a horrible idea, consider this simple fact. Research has now shown a link between a lack of sleep and heart disease. Those not getting enough sleep were much more likely to die from heart disease than their counterparts who were sleeping enough hours. There is a very real connection between quality sleep and being active.

Inactivity Is Damaging And In A Variety Of Ways

Today we are remarkably sedentary compared to just a generation ago. Not that long ago, most Americans lived on farms and as a result were performing a far amount of physical labor. Many of the modern medical conditions, such as a deficiency in vitamin D were almost unheard of as people were always outside. Only a few minutes outdoors allows the body to absorb enough vitamin D through the skin, but today people are becoming such "cave dwellers" that they actually have vitamin D deficiencies. There can be serious medical consequences to such a vitamin deficiency. Vitamin deficiencies can also take their toll on you mentally.

Thus, inactivity can decrease your overall health in ways that are not readily obvious. Most people know by now that a lack of exercise can lead to less muscle and less cardiovascular fitness. But as it turns out, being less active can radiate out in other directions, for example, not getting enough sunlight and therefore, not getting enough vitamin D. Once again, it is important to underscore that, where one's health is concerned, everything is interconnected.

The facts are that being physically inactive opens one up to a host of injuries, illnesses and disease. A lack of physical activity can lead to a weakened immune system, which means more colds, flus, and potentially even a greater risk of diseases like cancer. There is a great deal of research being done on the health benefits of exercise on the brain. It appears that working out can actually help the brain grow new neurological connections. It is amazing, but it is true.

Exercise and Depression

One reason that people are often not as active as they should be is that they are depressed. Depressed people often lack motivation. Factoring in everything that we have covered in this chapter, it should be clear that avoiding depression is critical for getting in shape, staying active and achieving your goals.

The fact that working out releases endorphins and in the process make you feel good is another major reason why physical fitness should be a priority. The "runner's high" that people get from working out could serve as a very powerful tool in fighting your own depression, and thus, achieving your goals.

Some evidence even points to the fact that working out might prevent depression altogether. Since it is vital to avoid depression in order to be more active and achieve your dreams, how can you possibly pass on exercising? At this point, it is becoming rather clear that the answer is that you simply can't.

Meditation and the Power of Being Active

At first glance, meditation and being active seem like diametrically opposed concepts. After all, isn't meditation about sitting still? No doubt this is the case, but there is more to meditation that sitting still. Mediation can be used to clear the mind and make a person more focused. Further, mediation can be used to clarify one's thoughts and determine where one's priorities should be.

It is possible to use meditation as a way to zero in on your goals. The act of stripping away all the chaos of an average day leads most people who meditate to having more clarity in their decision-making processes. As a result, you should be able to focus in on taking the steps necessary to make sure that you are indeed more active and are engaged in the steps necessary to change your life, drop the pounds and achieve your goals. Meditation has been used for centuries because it works. Medical science is beginning to find that meditation can improve health and brain function.

Remember that stress hormone cortisol? Cortisol can be reduced through meditation. Anything that you can do to reduce your stress level will benefit you both in body and mind; it's that simple.

Too Much Of A Good Thing

It is important to take a moment and consider that one can be too active. Just ask any single soccer mom who is working two jobs if one can be too active. Not having anytime to unwind or relax is also a serious problem as well, and it is a problem that must be guarded against. People can bury themselves and work and all sorts of other activities only to see that their entire lives have passed them by. One never wants to be so overcommitted that he or she never has a moment to relax.

Constantly being under pressure means that the stress hormone cortisol will flood your system. One of the impacts of cortisol, and one of the reasons you wish to avoid it, is that cortisol can make you gain weight. Thus, there is a connection between stress and weight gain. If you are looking to drop some pounds, then it makes good sense to reduce your stress level as well. Being overcommitted and pulled in too many directions could seriously impact all of your goals.

A smart move is to stop and evaluate how you spend your time. You should do this whether you think you are overcommitted or not. Evaluate how you spend your day and how you could make changes that would enable you to manage your time better. Time management might not be the sexiest term in history, but the facts are that time management is key for those looking to be active and make the most out of their time.

Tips For Time Management and Getting Active

- The first step in time management is to evaluate how you spend you time. You can start with a daily log of what you are doing hour-by-hour.

- Take your daily log of what you are doing hour by hour and look for wasted time. Everyone needs to relax but if you are spending too much time surfing the web or watching television, well, that is a problem. You want to be active!

- Commit yourself to new activities. Zero in on things that you like to do and join with friends or groups that will help keep you on target.

- Set aside a block of time for exercise and use it! Yes, this can be easier said that done. But most of us are creatures of habit. Once we have developed a new habit it is easier to stick with it.

- Reward yourself for good behavior. If something works then why not use it? Most of us like gifts and rewards and people simply do not reward themselves enough. If you have met your exercise and activity goals for a long enough period of time then maybe you've earned a reward.

Getting Active and Managing Stress

Stressed out people don't make the best decisions. We've all made poor decisions due to the fact that we were stressed out. It is important to stay calm, focused and happy when you are getting active, dropping some pounds and achieving your goals. Everything is very much connected. With this in mind, take steps to manage your stress so that you can stay focused and be active. If you keep your stress level low, you will realize the importance of exercise and the importance of being active.

Here are a few steps you can take to help you manage your stress.

1. Get a massage. Many shy away from massages because of the expense or time requirement. But for those looking to get fit and drop some pounds an

occasional massage is a good step in the right direction. Massages release stress and can help muscles with healing. It is believed that massage can help rid your body of cortisol!

2. Improve your diet. By eating higher quality foods you will feel better. Avoid foods high in chemicals and preservatives, and gravitate toward whole foods and organic if possible. Try it for a few weeks and you will be surprised how much better you feel.

3. A lack of sleep will cause your mind and body stress. Make sure you get enough sleep, even if you have to skip something else.

4. Drink plenty of water. Dehydrated people often do not make proper decisions. So drink plenty of water and avoid toxic drinks such as soft drinks.

5. Take a walk. While this one may sound way too simple taking a walk can do wonders for reducing your stress levels. Also taking a walk can get your outdoors where you can get some precious vitamin D.

Review This Chapter!

If you ever feel that your motivation for getting more active is starting to wane, simply review this chapter. Outlined in this chapter are numerous reasons why being physically fit is a must for anyone who is looking to drop pounds and keep those pounds off.

Every action that you take on your body is connected in some fashion. Keep this principle of interconnectivity in mind as you try and become more active. Realize that whatever impacts your outlook and attitude may very well impact how motivated you are to be physically active.

Chapter 11

STRETCHING

*"Blessed are the flexible, for they shall not
be bent out of shape." —Author Unknown*

Stretching

Life is busy, and as a result, it can be quite difficult to find time to work out. Yet, as we have covered in previous chapters, in order to get fit one must get active and stay active. Stretching most definitely emphasizes the staying active part of the equation. Think about it, if you are injured, you are out of the workout game. If you are unable to workout, then you are unable to drop pounds and meet your fitness goals. In short, not getting injured is a very big deal. Anything that you can do to prevent injury is a must.

Yet, avoiding injury has wider implications as well. If you have an injury, you are likely to be unhappy or at least not quite as happy as you should be or could be. Anyone who has ever "blown out" his or her back definitely understands how important it is to avoid injury. An injury such as a severe back injury can make the simplest of activities something of a nightmare. Getting out of bed becomes a painful ordeal, and even going to the washroom can be quite unpleasant!

While it may be obvious it does bear repeating that avoiding injury is a key part component in staying healthy and achieving your goals, including dropping a few pounds. Often this element of fitness is overlooked but it shouldn't be. Where fitness and reaching your goals are concerned everything is interconnected. If you are injured you are much more likely to be less motivated and may even become depressed.

An injury that occurs as a result of working out can be a tough one mentally as you might feel foolish for getting injured. Many people who exercise a good deal get injured through carelessness and those are the worst injuries psychologically. One way to avoid injuries of this nature is to take your pre-workout and post-workout routine seriously.

The Pre-Workout Ritual-Don't Get Injured

1. Make sure you are properly hydrated. As we have already pointed out in this book, most people don't drink enough water. Skip the weird waters that put chemicals into the mix, and just drink water.

2. Carry your water in a stainless steel bottle. In a word, it's worth the money. Plastic bottles have harmful plastics and chemicals in them that can have a wide range of negative effects. You don't need this. Spend a little extra on a stainless steel bottle. It's worth every penny.

3. Make sure you have enough calories in your system for a workout. There is nothing sadder, scarier or just plain weirder than watching someone pass out during a workout.

4. While on the subject of passing out during a workout, make it a ritual before every workout to remind you not to overdo it. This is a very important point. Remember if you are injured, you will make little or no progression toward your fitness goals.

5. Are you wearing the proper clothing? This is especially important for runners where shoes are concerned. A poorly fitting pair of athletic shoes can cause injury.

6. Consider your environment. Another aspect of your pre-workout ritual should be to consider your environment. Are you working out or exercising in a safe area? Paranoia can keep people from living their lives. But running through a sparsely populated area at five a clock in the morning just isn't bright. Remember, you have nothing to prove.

7. Part of your pre-workout ritual should include reminding yourself not to try and impress anyone. This includes you! Do not try and impress yourself or those around you. Once more if you are injured you cannot drop those pounds!

8. Are you focused enough to workout? This is a very important question and should not be taken lightly no matter how you are exercising. If you are lifting weights you can get hurt and seriously. If you are jogging, a car can hit you, for example. You get the point. You need to make sure that your head is in the game. Avoiding injury is a must in achieving your goals. Always stop before a workout and evaluate your mental preparedness.

9. Another part of your pre-workout ritual should be to determine if you are fit to workout. Many people simply will ignore this point and workout whether they feel up to it or not. Often this is done out of ego and its simply not prudent. If you are feeling under the weather your immune system needs the energy you would otherwise expend exercising and recovering afterwards. Weight-lifting means breaking down muscle and rebuilding that muscle takes a good deal of energy and valuable nutrition. If you are sick, you are out of commission.

10. Stretching is your friend. Stretching can help your body in a variety of ways. Often people think of stretching as something that they do before a workout, but as you will learn in this chapter stretching should be done at various points throughout the day.

Types of Stretching

One of the best ways to avoid injury is stretching. Over the centuries, a variety of forms of stretching have been developed. Stretching allows one to avoid injury well in advance and should be thought of as more than just a pre-workout precaution. Incorporating stretching into your lifestyle and routine is a way of increasingly blood flow to your muscles and increasingly flexibility as well. There are many ways to approach stretching but for our purposes we will look at a few of the most common types of stretching.

Yoga

When many people hear the word "stretching," one of the first associations that pops into their minds is often yoga. Yoga, originally developed in India, has been practiced for thousands of years, roughly 5,000 in fact. In the last few decades, this ancient health practice has undergone a period of wide scale discovery in the West. It is common now to find yoga studios in all part of the country, and in certain cities you may find dozens of yoga studios competing for attention.

Many mistakenly believe that if they are regularly attending yoga classes or practicing yoga that they are giving their bodies enough exercise. There is no doubt that yoga is one of the best physical activities that one can do for overall health; however, it is not a replacement for resistance training or cardiovascular training.

Breathing

Often overlooked, as a benefit of practicing yoga is the fact that it can help one learn valuable breathing techniques. Yoga focuses on proper breathing, and if you don't think proper breathing is important just ask an athlete or a woman in labor. Getting lots of oxygen into the body is critical for overall health and clear thinking.

After all, your brain needs oxygen to thrive and you need a clear head to make proper decisions. This means if you are stretching via yoga, you will also have the extra benefit of working on your breathing. Getting more oxygen into your body will also serve to real your mind and your muscles. It's a win-win!

Yoga and Flexibility

Yoga can do wonders for improving muscle strength and can even improve muscle and tendon strength, stamina and toughness, but only to an extent. As mentioned earlier in this book, yoga has been shown as an effective way to reduce stress levels. Like meditation, yoga may reduce the one's levels of stress hormones.

Even a quick look at the basic yoga poses should be enough to convince anyone that yoga can lead to greater flexibility. Stretching through yoga is no doubt one of the most effective ways of stretching, and if yoga becomes a major part of one's health care regiment, injuries from pulled muscles should be dramatically decreased.

Yoga and Safety

A word of caution concerning yoga: Like so many other practices, yoga has different levels of difficulty. It is only prudent to start off slowly, and then move to more advance poses over time. Also power yoga has been known to occasionally get someone hurt. Some of the more advanced poses could also easily lead to injury. This is, of course, the exact opposite of what we are attempting to accomplish. Thus, remember; start off slowly with any stretching you are doing. This means no head stands Mr. and Mrs. Overachiever!

Yoga and Achieving Your Goals

Yoga can certainly help you achieve your goals and help you lose some pounds. Staying focused, calm and clear headed is an aspect of dropping weight and achieving one's goals that is often overlooked. Yoga can help calm the mind much like meditation. It can also improve flexibility, thus meaning fewer injuries. As we have mentioned, yoga can even help teach proper breathing techniques. In short, yoga can do much more than just improve flexibility. There are even some early studies showing that yoga may help fight cancer and other diseases. With all of this in minds it is clear that yoga is far more than a system of stretching.

Pilates

Less known than yoga is Pilates, but the Pilates system has a good deal to offer as well. Pilates focuses a great deal on not just stretching muscles but increasing muscle strength, especially in the core muscles. Since we spend so much time in a seated position, our core muscles are simply not as strong as we would like them to be. Pilates is one of way of dealing with this lack of core strength.

Joseph Pilates developed the Pilates method during World War I as a new approach for rehabilitating injured soldiers. Like yoga, Pilates also focused on flexibility and breathing as well, but unlike yoga, Pilates uses a variety of instruments in order to help followers of Pilates achieve results. Strength building, flexibility and posture alignment are all major focal points for Pilates.

Those who are looking for a way to increase flexibility while increasing strength at the same time may want to consider Pilates. For this reason, Pilates has a good deal to offer especially from the perspective of time management.

Basic Stretching

Yoga and Pilates are both great. Both offer those who practice these systems a way to stretch and receive additional benefits at the same time. Yet for those who opt to just stretch, there are lots of stretching options ranging from the simple to the more advanced. Simply touching your toes and holding the pose is a great stretch for the back and hamstrings, for example.

In this era of the Internet, finding great stretching exercises is only a few clicks away. There is quite literally an abundance of websites that clearly show how to perform a variety of stretches. However, one should keep a few factors in mind whether performing stretches from a book or found on a website.

Important Stretching Tips

1. Does the stretch look too difficult or too extreme? If you are just beginning to stretch after years or even months of not stretching, don't push it.

2. Does the stretch look safe? If a stretch looks to extreme just skip it! Why risk injury while stretching?

3. Make sure you stretch your entire body. Not stretching your entire body is much like going to the gym and only working out your upper body. It makes zero sense and you shouldn't do it.

4. If you feel any pain stop! This point is so very important. The idea of "no pain-no gain" is for crazy people. Your goal is to avoid injury and stretching is supposed to help you avoid injury not cause it.

5. Make sure you are properly hydrated before stretching.

The Risk of Overstretching

Have you ever heard of someone being injured through overstretching? It most definitely occurs. Stretch too much and you can hurt yourself. Since our goal is to make sure you are healthy and able to do what is necessary to shed pounds, we should take a moment and address the importance of taking stretching slowly.

If you feel burning or tingling, just stop and don't try to force the muscle. Feeling your muscles stretch is one thing, as that is what you want to feel. However, feeling a strong tug on your muscle in another issue altogether and is something you want to avoid. Remember overstretching can cause more harm than good.

Stretching And Starting Slowly

A lot of times we all have a tendency to try and do too much, too quickly. Just as this attitude can be dangerous with weight lifting or jogging, it can be dangerous with stretching as well. Constantly remind yourself that there is no competition where stretching is concerned. The goal is to get more flexible at a healthy pace, not to see how quickly you can bend yourself into a pretzel!

If you haven't been physically active or haven't stretched in quite some time, start slowly. Remember, there is no one to impress. Give your muscles a chance to adapt stretching. Stretching should feel good and easy. If it feels difficult, you feel pain or are having trouble breathing, then you are either stretching too vigorously or there is some other problem. Back off immediately, and consider consulting your physician.

Your Stretching Environment

Sometimes you will want to do basic stretches when you are "out and about," and we will cover that soon. However, when you are engaged in more vigorous stretching, find a comfortable place with as few distractions as possible. When you are stretching being shocked or suddenly distracted can lead to injury. This can happen if you suddenly jump or twist in the wrong direction. Children and animals suddenly running into the room, for example, could be an issue. Try and cultivate as safe of a stretching area as possible.

When you are stretching in public, such as in a health club, yoga studio or gym, try to find a safe area where you are unlikely to bump into anyone or get in anyone's way. Remember the goal is always to avoid injury. If you are going to a class, simply leave yourself 5 extra minutes for this stretching.

Stretching is also a great time to calm and center your mind and focus on what you want. When you stretch, just breathe in and out and practice your visualizations. You may even want to look at your vision board when you are stretching. Think about the new body you will have and how good you will look. Imagine the fresh fruits and vegetables that you will be eating which will provide nutrients to your body. These quiet moments can be very powerful and effective at manifesting your goals and desires.

Where To Stretch

Some places are obvious places to stretch, but in order to improve your health and increase your flexibility you should find other places to stretch as well. It might be obvious to stretch before you workout whether that is at home or at the gym. Yet you should look for other places and ways to stretch.

Places To "Sneak In" Stretching

1. Work is a great place to sneak in some stretching, and you should every single chance you get. Sitting at a desk or lifting boxes all day can really cause muscles to tighten up. Taking a few moments and stretching your body so that the muscles can elongate can leave you feeling refreshed and more alert as well.

2. Also if you have ever had any back problems or suffer from neck and shoulder tension, taking a moment to stretch at work can work wonders to help reduce the occurrences and severity of these problems. There are many stretches specially designed for stretching where one does not even have to leave their desk.

3. Stretching in the car is a great idea. Of course, you want to be quite certain that you are not driving while stretching. However, when you are stuck in traffic or waiting at a red light, why not stretch? Learn some basic stretches that can be done in the car to help reduce your stress level. As we all know, being stuck in traffic can be very stressful. Stretching can help release some of that muscle tension. You can stretch all you want in the car and most likely the other drivers won't even notice!

4. Releasing stress can be very important while traveling. Learning some basic stretches is a good idea for anyone who travels. Find stretches that you can do while seated in an airplane or waiting in line.

Ways Of Incorporating More Stretching Into Your Life

1. Joining a gym and hiring a trainer is a great way to make sure you are stretching more. However, not all trainers are created equal or are even qualified. It is a bad sign if your trainer looks like he or she spends more time on the couch than at the gym. If you hire a trainer and they are not focused on you and what you are doing, then drop them immediately. And

don't give their feelings a second thought. Your trainer is not your friend; they are your trainer.

2. Have a workout partner and remind each other to stretch.

3. Pick a form of martial arts to study. This tip is for those who have been working out for a while. Martial artists and those who study martial arts are usually quite flexible. Studying a martial art, because the martial arts demand flexibility, is a good way to make sure you are flexible.

4. Join a yoga studio.

5. Take Pilates classes.

6. Set aside a time everyday for stretching, even if its only five minutes.

7. Set aside a few minutes a day at work for stretching. Again, just a few minutes can work wonders.

8. If necessary by a small alarm to remind you to stretch. Sometimes such steps are necessary and you shouldn't be afraid to take them.

9. Give yourself a reward if you meet your stretching goal. Just don't make that reward a high-calorie, high-fat snack.

10. Find a bunch of good websites and books dedicated to stretching. More than likely you will find some stretches that you like so much that you will want to do them each and every day!

Don't Overlook Stretching

Stretching is often overlooked in the fitness equation as weight lifting and cardiovascular activities receive all the "press" and attention. Yet the fact is that stretching can keep one healthy and avoid injury. Serious athletes know the value of stretching. If you ever watch athletes before a game, you often see them stretching and with good reason. They have learned from years of experience that not stretching can cause injury. They have learned from observing cause and effect as well as hearing from other athletes, coaches and trainers that stretching prevents injury.

> ... stretching can keep one healthy and avoid injury.

Just because you have never had an injury before does not mean you are immune. Even the strongest, most physically gifted athletes can get and do get injured. Stretching can help avoid injury and its benefits and preventive prowess should be taken seriously.

Chapter 12

EXERCISE

*"To keep the body in good health is a duty... otherwise we shall
not be able to keep our mind strong and clear." —Buddha*

We have already gone over the benefits of exercise quite a bit in this book.
It does not take a genius to understand that exercising helps keep pounds off and
helps our bodies stay fit and healthy. Exercising uses our muscles. This process takes
energy, which is taken from fat and glycogen. Yes, our fat is burned for fuel during
exercise. Even small children know that exercising can lead to weight loss. However,
we wanted to take this chapter and explore some practicalities to exercising, as well
as more suggestions for integrating it into your routine.

Most experts recommend a combination of exercises for losing weight. Weight
training, aerobic exercise and cardio workouts typically burn fat the fastest. When
we build muscle through weight training, we can burn energy even when we are at
rest. Aerobic and cardio workouts speed up our metabolism. This kind of exercise
also speeds up our metabolic rate is extremely important in that it helps us lose
weight quickly.

One problem that a lot of people have with exercise is that they overcommit to a
workout program that is really either too hard or will take up too much time in their
life. Although initially they have the best intentions, within a few weeks or a few
months they fall off track and then give up forever. It is important to find exercise
that you can integrate into your routine, hopefully, for good.

If you are unsure where you fall in regards to your physical fitness level, there
are a few easy ways to find out. Now remember that your goals for what you want to
achieve with your level of physical activity should always be your own. Remember

one of the first rules to the Law of Attraction is to determine what YOU want. This means that you shouldn't have to feel as though you should follow whatever exercise goals your friends have, a book you read suggests or a personal trainer tells you is necessary.

Physically fit means different things to different people. The main way to determine your immediate level of physical fitness needs is to look at the obvious. Do you easily get out of breath? Can you walk a mile without getting winded and exhausted?

If you really want to figure out what technically your level of physical fitness is, there are a few tests you can try. There is the Army's Fitness Test, for example, which breaks down standards for sex and for age. It then gives you corresponding tests and activities based upon these guidelines.

You could also determine your level of weight you potentially need to lose according to the BMI or Body Mass Index. The BMI simply has you add your weight and height into a formula. It then tells you if you are in the obese, overweight, normal or underweight category. You can find out your BMI score easily by just searching on Google "BMI." There are a wide variety of websites that will allow you to determine your Body Mass Index. It doesn't hurt to take a moment out and find where you fall on the BMI.

Another easy way to determine your current level of fitness is to test your pulse rate. A resting pulse rate of 60 beats per minute to 80 beats per minute is generally considered normal. During exercise, you can stop and take your pulse to make sure that you are in the correct zone. Once you have determined your pulse you can either increase or decrease the level of intensity of your workout.

Your target heart rate during a workout depends on your age to a certain degree as well as your current level of fitness. Where a 20 year old should be looking for a target heart rate between 100 and 170 beats a minute a 60 year old would want to have a target heart rate between 80 and 130 beats per minute. If you want to find out the perfect target heart rate for you, go and talk to your doctor.

Once they have figured out their target heart rate, many people use a heart rate monitor during their workouts to help them stay in the zone. You can buy a heart rate monitor for anywhere between $25 and $100.

Find Exercises that are Fun for You

There are a wide variety of types of exercises that you simply may not have thought of. Many of these exercises are also very social. For example, why not join a sports league where they play sports like softball, volleyball or soccer? As we have discussed, there is nothing wrong with getting into playing a sport you enjoyed as a child. These three sports are examples of how you can get exercise and also have a great deal of fun at the same time.

These sports are also excellent in that they get you working as a team and feeling comradeship. So many people feel isolated and alone these days, and so team sports can be a great fit not only to add exercise but also to add some fun and excitement into your day.

Another great idea for keeping exercising fun is to change the types of exercises you try. Now is the time to look into sports or activities that you always thought might be fun but never tried. In many regions, you can also find clubs or groups for people interested in a particular type of exercise. This makes exercising even more fun because you get to go out there and meet new people.

One great resource for finding people interested in particular sports or activities is www.meetup.com. Just type in your region and area and you will immediately start getting invitations for events going on. It's also a great way to make yourself feel very popular!

Here are some ideas for specific exercises that most people find to be a lot of fun.

1. **Hiking**

    Most areas have hiking trails where you can get out in natural settings and get some good walking done. Hiking can be much better than regular walking because you get to increase your endurance going up and down hills. You also often get to see some amazing scenery in the process. If you don't know about the hiking opportunities in your area, see if you can find a guidebook of trails in the library or on Amazon.com. You may be amazed at all the beautiful trails that are only a short distance away from you.

    Hiking is a great activity to sync up with the Law of Attraction. You get to do some great thinking or meditative walking when you are out on the trail. There is nothing to make you feel better about the possibilities of your current goals and desires than hiking to the top of a mountain or hill and looking out upon the horizon. Standing there, looking at the view, you can really cement your views that anything is possible and the future is wide open for you.

2. **Rock climbing**

    Rock climbing is a great activity and sport that you may have never thought of trying. If you live in a region that has mountains, you can actually get out there in nature and relate one on one with the terrain. Rock climbing can build strength, endurance, and flexibility.

However, even if you don't live near mountains you can still go rock climbing. Even if you do live near mountains, you may want to check out an indoor rock gym for practice or for when the weather is not conducive to going outdoors. Most cities and towns have rock-climbing gyms where people can try their hand at rock climbing. One of the great bonuses to rock climbing is that it is a physical as well as a mental challenge. Indoor rock climbing gyms also offer the basic instruction you need in the way of tying knots and using the safety harnesses.

Many people find that rock climbing is a great way to gain more confidence. There is nothing like looking at a big mountain that seems difficult to conquer, and then knowing that you did indeed conquer it yourself! The climbing itself also requires balance and coordination, so there are skills that will also be built up in the process.

3. **Winter Sports**

Many people get reclusive about their exercise during the winter and tend to stay indoors. However, in the winter, a whole realm of fun sports activities await you. Of course, there is skiing, which is great exercise and also a blast. Skiing can tone your entire body and is a fantastic cardio workout. It also is good for your heart muscles. Other winter sports include snowshoeing, cross-country skiing and snowboarding.

Snowshoeing offers a great aerobic workout. You get completely immersed in nature and burn lots of calories in the process. Snowshoeing is also much easier to learn than skiing or snowboarding. You can also rent the snowshoe equipment for fairly inexpensive rates.

Cross-country skiing is another great form of exercise. It also burns more calories than any other sport at the competitive racing level. Competitive cross-country skiers burn 900-1100 calories per hour. Regular recreational cross-country skiing burns about 600 per hour. Compare this amount of calories with that of speed walking at 400 calories burned per hour. Cross-country skiing has the leg up. This sport is very low-impact and is often considered to be one of the healthiest sports around.

Cross-country skiing is a total body workout. Have you ever seem people working out on Nordic trainer machines? That is why! Cross-country skiing gives you the pulling and pushing motion that is great for your body. It is not too taxing for any one muscle in your body, so you can do it for hours and hours on end. Also your heart rate speeds up, and you can keep it at this level for hours without taxing yourself too much. This activity is also great for the lungs because they must keep up with the increased respiration.

4. Dance

Dance is one of those activities that more commonly falls into the bracket of fun than it does exercise. However, dancing is an excellent form of cardiovascular exercise. People of all ages can find good venues to go out and dance on a Friday or Saturday night. Just think about the type of music you enjoy most, and then find a place where you can go ahead and dance to your favorite tunes. There are even dance venues geared towards seniors. One of the reasons that dance is so good for you is that it increases muscle tone, coordination, as well as energy levels. Dance is also a great stress reducer.

It doesn't even have to be dancing at nightclubs, there are classes around the world that teach people a variety of dance steps including Ballroom dancing, Salsa dancing, square dancing, belly dancing etc. Dancing also provides a great social component. With some dances you need to have a partner and work collaboratively with him or her. With other types of dancing you can feel the group energy and positivity. It is inspiring to be in an environment where everyone is happy, moving and having fun.

Also quite a few gyms offer aerobic exercise dance classes. Aerobic dance combines dance steps with more traditional forms of exercise. There may be kicks, jumping jacks and grapevines within the dance. Some aerobic dance classes integrate different types of ethnic styles such as African dance or Latin dance. You can also find hip-hop dance classes in many areas.

Here are some types of dance you could try that you may not have thought of:

- Belly Dancing
- Salsa
- Flamenco
- Jazz
- Tap Dancing
- Square Dancing
- Folk Dancing
- African Dance
- Zumba
- Swing
- Line Dancing
- Modern Dance

Enjoy the Social Aspect of Exercise

Many people have found that making exercise social is a great way to stay consistent and not miss any exercise dates. If you have already told a friend that you will be there, you are more likely to show up and have a positive attitude. After all, you know you will get to catch up with your friend and joke around while the exercise takes place. So how can you make exercise social? This could be as simple as scheduling a long hike, a jog or a bike ride with a friend. In fact, this sort of exercise routine can be substituted for something like going for a beer or going out to dinner. It will benefit both you and your friend.

One of the reasons that people like to workout in gyms so much is because of the social benefit of working out with other people. There is a major advantage to getting out of your house and picking up on other people's energy and good attitude about working out. There is nothing wrong with working out at home with an exercise video, but you could definitely miss out on the social component.

On the other hand, if you can't afford a gym membership, why not invite a friend or two to your house to follow an exercise video with you? Working out at home does have its benefits. For example, you don't need to care what you wear and you don't lose travel time getting to and from the gym location. There are also a lot of great yoga videos that you could try. Working out at home with friends can work great if you want to switch out the videos for new ones every couple of weeks. Have each friend bring one video of his or her choice each week.

Many people who have dogs are in luck, because dogs offer us a constant good and social reason to get some exercise. Your dog is always in the mood for exercise. In fact, if he doesn't get outside and take a walk everyday it is actually bad for his health. There really isn't much that your dog loves more than getting outside with you and taking a walk. Watch how much it means to your dog just to get out there and start moving his or her body.

Dogs also have a constant love of exploration. Every day your dog gets outside there is something new to enjoy. Try to take a hint from your dog and get into the same mind frame. This fits extremely well with the Law of Attraction. Every day there is something new to appreciate outdoors. In fact, getting out there and being able to walk is something to appreciate in and of itself.

We often recommend for those who are having trouble getting motivated to get outside and walk to just get a dog. Your dog will definitely prove to be a great inspiration to keep you on track. He will always be ready to get up and go. Try to cultivate much the same attitude when it comes to working out!

You can also just go out in the park with a friend and throw around a Frisbee. Chasing a Frisbee always feels way more like fun than a solid form of exercise. If you don't have a friend handy that wants to play Frisbee, why not throw one to your dog. Your dog is always up for exercise. In fact, having your dog with you tends to make most anything you do more fun.

Fitting Exercise into Your Day-to-Day Schedule

One of the things that thinking about the Law of Attraction will do is keep your mind open to new possibilities. In fact, it is common that once you have realigned your mind to be more positive, creative solutions may start coming to you automatically.

One of the benefits to this is that you will more than likely begin to think of ways to incorporate exercise into your day that never occurred to you before.

If you have an office job, there are plenty of creative ways to fit exercise into your day. Here are some ideas that you may not have thought of:

- **Park your car further away**

    One very easy idea is to park your car a further distance away in the parking lot so you walk to and from your car. If you take the subway, you could also consider getting off of the subway one stop early and walking the rest of the way to work. This very easy step can add up to a lot more exercise over the course of a month or even a year,

    You can also do the same thing when you go grocery shopping. Park your car farther away than you need to and then carry the grocery bags all the way to your car. (Of course, your amount of groceries must be within reason. You may not want to try this if you are carrying 2 weeks worth of groceries for a family of 4.)

- **Take a 5 or 10-minute walk on your lunch break.**

    It is easy to take a short walk on your lunch break for extra exercise. You may even be able to get a co-worker to walk with you to make it more social. Another benefit to taking a short walk is that you get some fresh air and sunlight. Sunlight has been shown to increase our levels of Vitamin D. Vitamin D is needed to regular our body's functioning.

    Often people get SAD or Seasonal Affective Disorder because they have not gotten enough sunlight in the wintertime. SAD can cause depression, lack of energy and agitation. However, increased levels of Vitamin D have been shown to improve mood during the winter. This is an additional benefit that will go along with your exercise break.

- **Do some stretches at your desk.**

    We already covered this in the stretching chapter. Why not do some simple stretches at your desk? Assuming that you are not getting in anyone's way, feel free to do some leg lifts and toe touches.

- **Take the stairs.**

    Why lose valuable exercise taking the elevator, when you get in some cardiovascular activity taking the stairs? People who take the stairs up and down to their office each day are doing themselves a major service. Whenever you have the chance to take advantage of a chance to use your body to get in a little workout, you should take it.

    If you want to take the "take the stairs" idea even a step further, why not carry a heavy bag up and down with you? One day you could try taking two stairs at a time. Or you could try timing yourself to see how fast you can go up and down the stairs. You could even increase the weight in the bag every day with an additional book. This sort of training is easy free and can be fun too when you make it into a game for yourself.

Avoiding Injury

Here is another good reason not to push yourself too hard during a workout. If you do, you could put yourself at a risk for injury. This is especially if you are accustomed to leading a sedentary lifestyle. If you all of a sudden push yourself to the max, you could potentially injure yourself. Once you have injured yourself, you could set back your goals and plans considerably.

It only makes sense to take proper measures to exercise in a safe way. One important guideline is to always drink plenty of water when you exercise. If you get dehydrated, it can get dangerous for you. You could get disoriented and potentially make an accidental lapse of judgment. Another important guideline is to stop exercising if you happen to feel pain. When you feel pain your body is really telling you to stop and slow down. Pay attention to that little voice in your head when it tells you that you have had enough.

Another aspect of your exercise regime that you should not overlook is your flexibility. As we discussed in our chapter on stretching, it is really important to be flexible to move well and avoid injury. There are great exercises for becoming more flexible.

Also don't try too much too soon. Even if you have very extreme goals, you can achieve them with the Law of Attraction. For example, someone who has never hiked before may have the goal of hiking to the top of Mount Everest. However, without any training, he or she would be best advised not to try right away. If your goal was to fly, for example, we wouldn't really suggest that you try it right away either. However, remember don't try too much too fast. There is no one to try to impress. Slow and steady wins the race!

Chapter 13

THE TEN BEST SUPERFOODS

"It is wonderful, if we chose the right diet, what an extraordinarily small quantity would suffice." —Deepak Chopra

Modern science has certainly learned a great deal in recent years about the human body and how it responds to nutrition. Further, medical science has also learned a great deal about what kinds of impact different foods have on our body and even on dropping pounds. There can be no doubt that nutrition plays a role in weight loss. In fact, nutrition and how one deals with his or her food is the cornerstone of not only keeping thin, but of good health in general. The recent explosion in knowledge concerning what foods are best for human consumption gives new tools to those who are looking to keep healthy and fit.

By selecting the best of the superfoods, it is possible to give your diet, your health and your goals a jumpstart. The trick is to envision superfoods helping you reach your health and fitness goals. Don't be afraid to overhaul your diet and eating habits with these healthy and nutritious foods. Remember most of our

> ... envision superfoods helping you reach your health and fitness goals.

modern diets are often lacking and full of chemicals and preservatives. You can use superfoods as a tool towards better health and a slimmer waistline.

No doubt there are a great many foods that have been shown to be, well, super by modern science. In general, it makes sense to eat a variety of healthy foods, and by healthy we mean not from a prepared packages. As we discussed in the Food Choices chapter, it is best to stay away from highly processed foods. We will explore this a bit further in the next chapter entitled "10 Foods You Should Never Eat Again."

Some of the foods you are about to read about might be foods that you have either not eaten before, or have not eaten much of in the past. It is important that you give them a try and try to incorporate them into your regular diet because they are very good for you. Try to keep in mind that being overly picky or set in your dietary ways will not ultimately help you achieve your health and fitness goals.

In a sense, superfoods are a short cut towards eating healthy. If you are consuming all the foods on this list, then you probably are eating a healthy diet. Many of these foods are so nutritious and filling that they will quench your desire to eat too much. They will also get you inspired to eat more and more fresh, healthy food.

There are many foods that are worthy of being on a superfoods list. In fact, what the ten best superfoods are which are definitively the best vary a bit from expert to expert. But for our purposes, the one's that work best with a weight-loss program have been highlighted. Further, foods were selected that are readily available and can usually be found in one's local grocery store.

Garlic

Some of you might be wondering how garlic made it onto the superfoods list. How can I get full eating garlic? The bottom line is that garlic is such an amazing food that everyone should be eating it all the time. For thousands of years, garlic has been prized for its ability to fight off colds and disease. But it's only been in the last few decades that modern science has been able to unlock some of garlic's various secrets.

Garlic has an array of powerful chemicals that serve to help defend the human body against a host of diseases. Chemicals in garlic have anti-viral, anti-fungal and anti-bacterial properties that have been clinically shown to work at fighting off infections and diseases across the board. Now you might be tempted to think that this has nothing to do with losing weight, but your wrong. If you keep getting run down with colds or the flu, you will not be able to stay on your diet or work out. Thus, for anyone looking to lose weight, stay in shape and be healthy, garlic is your friend. In fact, garlic is one of your very best dietary friends in the world.

These facts concerning garlic are impressive. Yet, garlic it is a food that has even more to offer than its anti-bacterial, anti-viral and anti-fungal properties. Garlic is surprisingly nutritious as it has a great many vitamins and minerals. Many people are surprised to learn that garlic is actually rather high in vitamin C and vitamin B6, for example. Garlic has no less than fifteen major vitamins and minerals contained in its little bulbs. So when you are reaching for a clove of garlic, you are actually receiving a great deal of nutrition as well.

Studies are also showing that garlic can help your heart by addressing issues relating to high blood pressure. Garlic may even work to help prevent a variety of types of cancer. Recent studies are returning very strong indications that garlic can reduce the rates of some types of cancers by very large percentages.

Best of all, garlic is safe for most people to use. It makes all sorts of foods taste great. For anyone looking to drop pounds adding garlic is a wise move, as it will add tremendous flavor to any dish.

Five Ways To Get More Garlic In Your Diet

1. Feel free to seek out recipes that have lots of garlic in them. Cookbooks are loaded down with recipes that have lots of garlic. We have offered some of our favorites in the final chapters of this book.

2. Its easy to add chopped garlic to your salads and tasty as well.

3. Consider cooking more with garlic. After a while, you'll instinctively know just how much to add to make many dishes taste just great.

4. Garlic and soups work very well together.

5. Dishes like hummus are wonderful places to toss in garlic.

Blueberries

Much like garlic, blueberries should be seen as your friend. Blueberries have received significant attention in recent years for good reasons. Blueberries are simply brimming over with compounds that improve overall health.

Currently, there is a good deal of research being conducted into how blueberries can even work to protect overall brain health and may protect one's vision as well. In terms of nutrition the blueberry should be on everyone's plate.

Part of why blueberries make for such a fantastic weight-loss and nutrition food is that they give dieters so much for the calorie. Blueberries are so low in calories that you can almost eat as many as you feel like, the key word being almost. This tiny little superfood is also quite high in nutrition packing lots of vitamin K, manganese as well as vitamin C. Of course the nutritional values vary depending upon where the type of blueberry and where it is grown so make sure you check the label.

Five Ways To Get More Blueberries In Your Diet

1. The fact that blueberries freeze so well means that you can keep them on hand year round and use them whenever you want.

2. Blueberries work very well in juices and shakes as blueberries are naturally sweet. One each way to get more blueberries into your diet is to simply toss them into shakes.

3. Blueberries love taking a bath in oatmeal or cereal. You will find that blueberries in your oatmeal or cereal work very well.

4. Breakfast is a great time for incorporating this amazing little berry. Toss blueberries onto your pancakes the next time you make a stack.

5. If you keep frozen blueberries on hand, and you should, you can always have them as a snack or toss some on your plate any time of the day.

Walnuts

Somewhere along the way people started believing that all fat is bad fat. This is simply not the case. The human body needs a degree of healthy fat in order to be healthy and function properly. That stated, this does not mean that you run out and eat four steaks with a baked potato smothered in butter. The fats you are looking for are healthy fats. Nut, in general, can provide the human body with a good deal of healthy fats. Walnuts show some real promise in terms of how they can help human health over the long term. While walnuts are not a low-calorie food, in moderation, they are a good health food as they can help reduce hunger cravings and fat cravings.

The health benefits of walnuts are pretty substantial and while people have long known that walnuts were good for you it is only in recent years that we have begun to see what walnuts were "really made of." The humble walnut might not look like too much but it's really a major player in the health world.

Much of what makes walnuts such an excellent food is the fact that it is so high in omega-3 fatty acids. Omega-3 fatty acids are vital for brain health and also have some seriously anti-inflammatory punch. Studies also show that walnuts are great for the heart too. If you are still not convinced consider that walnuts are antioxidant rich as well.

Walnuts, like many of the other superfoods we are covering, are easy to buy, easy to store and easy to use. Here are few ways you can get more walnuts in your diet.

Five Ways To Get More Walnuts In Your Diet

1. Simply add a small handful of walnuts to your favorite salad. But remember walnuts, like most nuts are high in calories, so go easy. The only low-calorie nut is the chestnut.

2. Walnuts go great in all kinds of baked deserts and dishes like muffins. Throw in a few walnuts and your brain and heart will thank you.

3. Experiment with walnut friendly recipes. Walnuts are so versatile that you can find all sorts of recipes that have walnuts already incorporated as a major component.

4. Tossing in a few walnuts into your breakfast cereal, oatmeal, pancakes or whatever other breakfast food you are having is a great way to start off the day.

5. Low-calorie walnut cookies!

Broccoli

Whenever anyone is referencing or discussing superfoods, broccoli should come up. Broccoli is most definitely one of the top, perhaps even the top, vegetable that one can eat. Eating broccoli is simply one of the best steps that you can take toward better health. In terms of weight-loss, broccoli is at the top of the list of foods that those who are looking to lose weight should be eating.

Broccoli is an impressively filling food that is very low in calories. Most people will probably become full long before they have consumed more than three or four hundred calories of this superfood. Now, remember, that is three or four hundred calories without butter, cheese or any other high-calorie topping added on!

What makes broccoli so amazing is that broccoli is a cancer fighting superfood. Broccoli is abundant in chemicals and enzymes that fight the growth and development of cancer cells. The nutrition in broccoli is another reason it is a winner. Just thirty calories of broccoli have about 150% of the RDA in vitamin C as well and decent numbers of about fifteen other major vitamins and minerals. Broccoli most definitely deserves to be on the superfood list, without a doubt.

Five Ways To Get More Broccoli In Your Diet

1. No crying if you don't like broccoli. This superfood is too good for you to pass on. If you are not adding raw broccoli to your salad, you should start doing so immediately!

2. If you don't own a juicer, consider purchasing one. A juicer is a fine investment in your health and will allow you to juice broccoli. This way you can blend broccoli in with other fruits and vegetables such as apples and carrots if you don't like the taste of broccoli.

3. Look for creative ways to steam broccoli for variety.

4. Consider adding a side of broccoli to your meals a couple of times a week.

5. Broccoli ice cream! Well, no not really, but try adding some broccoli on the side the next time you make scrambled eggs or an omelet. This actually works very well.

Wild Alaskan Salmon

Quality sources of protein are increasingly becoming an issue these days. It seems that everywhere you look there is another kind of scary story about the meat, poultry and fish that we consume. The truth of the matter is that we have to be more careful than ever about the animal protein that we consume. A good alternative is salmon, but it should be noted that not all salmon is the same.

Most fish has issues concerning contamination. This is a sad fact, but true. As a result of heavy metal contamination, it is smart to select wild Alaskan salmon over farmed salmon and Atlantic salmon. While not perfectly free of contaminants such as mercury, wild Alaskan salmon is, in general, safer than other salmons. The majority of all salmon sold is actually farmed salmon and farmed salmon has been tied to serious contamination issues. Farmed salmon should be avoided altogether.

Salmon is an excellent protein source for dieters in that it is a low-calorie, low-fat protein source that is high in protein and has a great deal of healthy fats. Just like walnuts contain high levels of omega-3 fatty acids the same can be said of salmon. Further, salmon is high in numerous vitamins, including vitamin D and several B vitamins and even has antioxidants. In terms of animal protein, salmon is a top pick.

Five Ways To Get More Salmon In Your Diet

1. Salmon is an easy food to incorporate into your diet. You can broil it or bake it like you would most other fishes. Just don't fry it!

2. Salmon can be a fine addition to a soup, such as miso soup.

3. Try salmon in a salad. Salmon salad works great with a little lemon.

4. Salmon can work for breakfast. Try tossing a little salmon in with your omelet or serve it on the side.

5. Grilling is something that should be done sporadically due to the carthogenic compounds produced during the grilling process. However, when you do grill, consider a piece of wild Alaskan salmon instead of a fatty burger.

Sardines

Yes, sardines. Many people may turn up their noses at these little fish, but the fact they are little is one of the reason that you should consider adding them to your weight-loss plan. Sardines, because they are smaller, are lower on the food chain. You've probably seen an animation or cartoon of bigger fish eating smaller fish. No doubt this is the case, and where your diet and health is concerned this is a pretty significant issue. The larger the fish the more likely it is that contaminants, such as heavy metals like mercury, are present in high numbers. Since sardines are lower on the food chain, they generally have less contamination and are safer to eat.

Like salmon and walnuts, sardines are high in omega-3 fatty acids, which are brain, and heart healthy fats that you want in your body. Sardines are low in calories but high in protein and also serve as a fine source of vitamin D and calcium.

The fact that sardines can be bought in the can means that you can always have them handy year round. You may not be familiar with sardines, but it the sardine is a very versatile fish and if you don't like the taste try finding a recipe that works for you.

Five Ways To Get More Sardines In Your Diet

1. Don't be afraid of a sardine stew. Find a good recipe and give it a try.
2. Grilled sardines, on occasion, are very tasty.
3. Toss a few sardines into your salad for a low-calorie protein.
4. Sauté some sardines with garlic, salt, pepper and red pepper. Serve this spicy mixture with some organic rice.
5. Look for recipes and experiment. Odds are you will be able to find all sorts of ways of swapping out sardines in the place of other animal proteins.

Green Tea

Green tea is another food that deserves to be on the superfoods list. Simply replacing coffee with green tea is a way to improve your overall health. Perhaps even replace one or two cups of your daily java fix with green tea to begin with, and then work up to a full switch.

The reason that green tea is such an impressive superfood is that it has no calories, yet is loaded with all sorts of wonderful compounds that can improve overall health. Hundreds, and that is no exaggeration, of studies by governments and universities around the world have concluded that green tea has the ability to fight cancers of various kinds and appears to fight off cavities as well. There is a powerful antioxidant in green tea, EGCG, which has a wide-variety of health benefits. Many of the claims that are being made about green tea are unproven, but enough has been proven about green tea to make it a worthy addition to the superfood list.

Green tea can help you lose weight in two ways. One, use green tea as a replacement for higher calorie drinks you might be consuming. Secondly, there is evidence that green tea speeds up one's metabolism.

Five Ways To Get More Green Tea In Your Diet

1. The easiest way for most people to get more green tea in their diet is to trade out a cup or two of coffee for green tea.

2. Set aside a meal or time of the day to drink green tea.

3. Green tea does have a good amount of caffeine; so don't drink it late at night.

4. Keep green tea bags in your desk at work. Better yet, keep a green tea bag or two on your desk to remind you to drink tea instead of coffee!

5. Buy a variety of green teas. Odds are you will find one that you really love and that will help you drink more green tea.

Eggs

Many might be surprised to see eggs on the superfood list. For years we've heard about how horrible eggs are for you. But an egg a day, if the rest of your diet isn't swimming in cholesterol, will probably only help you. That stated, if you have high cholesterol or serious health issues, you best check with your doctor before upping your consumption of eggs. Yet for most people an egg every day or every other day is not just fine, its good for you. Just opt for organic free range eggs whenever possible.

Eggs are a great weight-loss and diet food because they are low in calories and high in protein. It is important that you get enough protein when you are dieting. Eggs are a fine way to make sure that you do have enough protein in your diet. When one takes a careful look at how much nutrition is in an egg, eggs become even more impressive. Eggs are high in numerous B vitamins, phosphorus, vitamin A and choline. Choline, in particular, is very important for brain health. Eggs are also high in some key amino acids such as glutamic acid, an important neurotransmitter.

When buying eggs it is best to select free range, organic eggs. Many health experts feel that the eggs that come from large "egg factories" are often inferior to their free-range counterparts. In general, free range chicken also experience a dramatically superior quality of life, similar to what chickens experienced on the farms of past.

Five Ways To Get More Eggs In Your Diet

1. Eggs are an extremely easy food to work into your diet. Recipes abound for the wonderful egg. Find a good recipe book and you will find all sorts of ways to work in the egg.

2. Eggs go great in salads.

3. Eggs are a mainstay at the breakfast table. Consider bring the egg back to your breakfast table.

4. Don't exclude the egg from dinnertime. Why not try an egg on the side if your meal is lacking a protein?

Extra Virgin Olive Oil

Olive oil has been used for since ancient times, and this amazing food should still have a prominent place in the diets of most people today. Olive oil is of course very high in fat content. However, like walnuts, olive oil is considered to be a healthy fat. The fat in olive oil is monounsaturated, which is actually considered to be heart healthy.

The list of pros in favor of consuming olive oil is rather high. Olive oil, in addition to its quality fat content, is high in antioxidants, rich in both vitamins K and E and has an anti-inflammatory effect. However, it is essentially 100% fat, and with this in mind, one must use olive oil in a logical fashion. Yet, few foods can match olive oil for its overall health benefits.

Those looking to drop pounds should not forgo all fat from their diets. Incorporating healthy fat into your diet is a vital part of health. Olive oil is so good for you that it should play a role in your day-to-day diet and day-to-day dieting.

Extra virgin olive oil is easy to buy. In fact, it is one of the most commonly available cooking products out there. But make sure you buy only extra virgin olive oil, which is by far the highest quality.

Five Ways to Get More Extra Virgin Olive Oil In Your Diet

1. Keep your olive oil bottle out so that you can see it. This way you will remember to use your olive oil more regularly.

2. Olive oil is so easy to use. For example, simply toss a little olive oil onto a salad.

3. Olive oil can be used for cooking, but its best if you do not use it at temperatures above about 350 degrees.

4. Look for recipes that use olive oil. Greek and Italian foods are famous for using olive oil.

5. Foods like hummus make for an excellent medium in which to "sneak in" a little extra olive oil. Just remember not to add too much!

Black Beans

How has the simple black bean made it onto the superfood list? The answer is that black beans are readily available and extremely nutritious. Virtually any supermarket you enter will have black beans in some form or another and black beans are one seriously nutritious food. Black beans are rich in folate, calcium, iron, zinc, magnesium, protein and fiber. Depending upon the variation, black beans may have even more nutrition as well, including additional B vitamins and minerals such as molybdenum.

What black beans offers dieters for the calories makes it a superfood. The simple black bean is a great source of protein and fiber and this makes it a fantastic diet food. When considering superfoods that are great for dieters, it is important to look for foods that are filling and nutrition. There can be no doubt that black beans definitely meet those criteria.

Five Ways to Get More Black Beans In Your Diet

1. The versatility of black beans is part of the reason they must be considered a superfood. One easy way to get black beans in your diet is to incorporate them into foods such as tacos.

2. Adding black beans to salads is a smart way to add more protein to your average salad.

3. Black beans seem as though they were made for soups, so definitely consider adding some black beans to your next soup.

4. Black beans are, quite surprisingly, high in antioxidants. Consider adding black beans as a side dish whenever possible. Find several good standard side dish recipes that incorporate black beans.

5. Find recipes that call for black beans as the centerpiece and main attraction of the recipe and make those recipes a regular in your cooking repertoire.

Chapter 14

THE TEN FOODS YOU SHOULD NEVER CONSUME AGAIN

"Meanwhile, the chemical industry has mounted an aggressive campaign to discredit organic food. And without the knowledge or consent of most Americans, two-thirds of the products on our supermarket shelves now contain genetically engineered ingredients." —John Robbins

Ok, now that we have gone over ten superfoods for dieters, we are now going to discuss some foods that are so terrible for you, we want you to go ahead and put them on your list of foods to never eat again. Brace yourself, here they are: French fries, doughnuts, non-dairy products (creamers and ice cream toppings), bacon, cookies and crackers with transfats, soda, frozen dinners, diet soft drinks, fast food and movie theatre or microwave popcorn.

We understand that this might seem hard at first. Rule out a food for the rest of your life? How is this even possible? There are so many delicious foods in the world, how can I make a promise to restrict myself from one, never mind ten, forever? Perhaps some of the above-mentioned are your favorites and you cannot imagine life without them.

However, don't throw this book down in horror just yet. The fact of the matter is that we promise you that when you start to switch your diet over to fresh, nutritious wholesome foods, these 10 Foods we are about to describe will no longer seem so appealing. Your body will no longer crave these foods. In fact, if you eat them you very well may end up feeling sick and ruining your entire day.

Think back to our Food Choices chapter and how we discussed the Law of Attraction's relationship to food. Like attracts like. The more unhealthy foods you eat, the more you will want. Conversely, the more healthy nutritious foods you eat, the more healthy foods your body will crave. When you give that rule of thumb some real consideration, it only makes sense what you should be eating.

Part of the reason you think that you want these unhealthy foods is that you are used to eating them. It is like any addiction, when you literally feed the addiction; you want more of the drug. If you think that comparing unhealthy food to drugs is unreasonable, read on!

Soda

Soda is definitely one of the foods that you should avoid for life. The amount of sugar and caffeine in soda is really off the charts. We have discussed the importance of water and staying hydrated. What is really sad is when people substitute soft drinks for water when they are thirsty. Not only are you not giving your body the water it so desperately needs, you are giving it a host of chemicals and preservatives to try and eliminate. Your body needs water, but you are giving it no water and making it even harder to detoxify.

Additionally, soda has a bunch of chemicals and preservatives. Next time you have a soda, take a look at the ingredients. Do you recognize any of them? You probably don't. But soda's real problem is the sugar. High-Fructose corn syrup is a cheap form of sweetener. Sugar can lead to tooth decay. In fact, there have been a variety of studies linking tooth decay and soft drinks. The acid in soda can also harm tooth enamel. "Acid begins to dissolve tooth enamel in only 20 minutes," notes the Ohio Dental Association

Also there is the Phosphoric acid, which is ever present in carbonated drinks. Phosphoric acid has been shown to de-oxidizes blood. Also this chemical is difficult for kidneys to remove. It can also deplete the body of calcium leading to weaker bones. Not to mention there is tons of caffeine in soda, which can also be very harmful, especially to kids who may get addicted to caffeine early in life. A 1994 Harvard study showed than teenage girls who drank soda were five times more likely to suffer bone fractures.

You can remove rust with soda, seriously. Is this really something you should be drinking? According to HowToCleanAnything.com, Coke can clean a toilet if you let it sit for an hour. It can also remove rust from a car bumper and clean corrosion from battery terminals.

Diet Sodas

Ok, so the sugar in soda is bad. Well, what about artificial sweeteners then? How about a can of Diet Coke or Diet Pepsi? There is a lot of controversy around about exactly how safe artificial sweeteners like Sweet'N Low, NutraSweet and Spleda actually are. For example, many experts believe that when the artificial sweetener Asparatame is heated beyond 86 degrees it converts to formaldehyde. However, the FDA still reports that diet sodas are safe. On the other hand, people have talked about side effects firsthand including dizziness, headaches, and memory loss, to name a few. However, even if the artificial sweeteners aren't enough to dissuade you, there are other reasons not to drink diet sodas.

Prevention Magazine recently published an article called "Newest Soda Danger Discover the Dangers of Diet Soda" which said that diet soda may increase the risk of what is called "metabolic syndrome," which gives you fat, blood sugar issues and high cholesterol. According to a University of Minnesota study, people who drank a diet soda once a day had a 34% higher risk of metabolic syndrome.

Dr. Mercola published an article a few years ago called "Diet Sodas May Double Your Risk of Obesity." Apparently, according to researchers at the University of Texas, people are 65% more likely to be overweight if they drink one or more diet soda a day. If they drink more than 2 diet sodas, the chances that someone is overweight are even higher! This study speculates that people who drink diet sodas may seek to compensate with a high calorie food. Even though the tongue tastes a sweet drink, the brain may still feel that it requires calories.

Foods with Transfat

Foods with transfat are quite common in our grocery store. The most common items to contain transfat are things like cookies, crackers and bread. However, you eat transfat, you will gain more weight than you would if you were eating healthy fats. Just like all calories are not created equal, all fats are also not created equal.

So what is a transfat? A trans fat is the result of liquid oils that have solidified. You can find something like "partially hydrogenated soybean oil" on the label of your food because the process often includes partial hydrogenation, a process that uses hydrogen gas. Sometimes the labels will simply say 'shortening" or 'hydrogenated vegetable oil." Once oils have been partially hydrogenated, they are easier to transport and have a longer shelf life. Foods that have partially hydrogenated soybean oil in them are also said to taste and feel less greasy.

These saturated fats are bad for you. They can raise low cholesterol while lowering your good cholesterol. Saturated fats have also been shown to cause diseases like cancer. One Harvard nutrition expert even called trans fats "the biggest food processing disaster in US history."

Healthy fats that your body actually wants includes oils like olive oil and coconut oil, avocadoes, nuts, to name a few. When you replace transfats with healthy fats, you will be making your journey to health quicker and easier. Good fats, in fact, also provide benefits for the body. They can reduce cholesterol levels, and reduce inflammation, for example.

Fast Food

With your new eating habits and lifestyle, you are definitely going to want to forget that fast food exists. The reasons to avoid fast food restaurants are pretty extensive. If you want to understand some of these reasons in detail, we highly recommend the book Fast Food Nation by Eric Schlosser. In the book Schlosser goes into detail about the horrors of the fast food industry. For example, he covers how mistreated the animals are, how unsanitary the meatpacking plants can be, and even how many of the flavors we experience in fast food restaurants are actually just chemicals that food scientists replicate to taste like food.

Eating foods that contain chemicals which make them taste similar to real foods are a total 180 from eating fresh wholesome food. Many fast food restaurants simulate these flavors we love so that they can cut costs on the food. They have discovered that if they can use chemicals instead of fresh ingredients they will save on the bottom line.

Here are Some Other Reasons to Avoid Fast Food:
- The food contains high levels of fat, calories, sodium, sugar and cholesterol.
- The food at fast food restaurants is typically devoid of nutrients. This means that we will get filled up on food with little nutrition. As a result, we don't get the essential nutrition that our bodies actually need.
- Food high in cholesterol will clog the arteries.
- Food that is high in sodium can also cause health problems. Excessive sodium will cause the heart to pump harder, thus, increasing blood pressure. Heart disease and hypertension can be the end result of this process.

Unlike many diet advocates, we don't suggest even going into fast food restaurants for what they call a salad. The fact of the matter is that chemicals and preservatives are hidden in many of the foods that fast food restaurants call "healthy." Men's Health magazine recently published an article called "The 20 Worst Foods in America." Right on this list was a fast food restaurant salad. The On the Border

Grande Taco Salad with Taco Beef has 1450 calories. This is as many calories as many women eat in one whole day. Truly, it is better to avoid fast food restaurants altogether. If you are eating in a fast food establishment, it is way to easy to say, "I will just have a soda," or "I will just have a small order of fries."

Doughnuts

Ah, the doughnut. Doughnuts, while one of America's favorite foods, are also one of the worst. The interesting thing is that many countries around the world have their own version of the doughnuts. There are doughnuts in China, India, Japan and most of Europe. Everyone seems to love ring shaped fried fritters.

So what about our doughnuts in the United States? Unfortunately, the white sugar and white flour in doughnuts offer us no nutritional benefits whatsoever. Why would you want to eat something that offers no nutrition?

Another major problem with doughnuts is they typically have lots of trans fats and saturated fats. As we discussed, this bad fat can reduce the benefits of the good fats that you eat. Some doughnuts even have as much as 10 grams of fat! And if you fill your doughnut with cream, the fat level can double to 21 grams. If you are eating fruit filled doughnuts hoping to get a little fruit into the mix, think again. Usually doughnuts are filled with chemicals made to taste like fruit.

French Fries

When many people hear that French fries are foods that they should avoid for the rest of their lives, they think, "French fries? Aren't potatoes healthy and natural? French fries couldn't be that bad, could they?" You may also think, "But aren't they French? French people are some of the healthiest people on earth. What about all those beautiful French models in perfect shape?"

The fact of the matter is that French fries have very little to do with potatoes. Also white potatoes are not really an extremely healthy food. If you want a potato, a yam or sweet potato is a much better choice. The white potato is high on the glycemic index. The glycemic index often called the GI measures how fast our food turns into sugar. If a food is high on the GI, this means that it quickly converts to sugar in our bloodstream. This means that they are likely to get stored as far if we don't use these carbs right away for energy. There is nothing wrong with having white potatoes every now and then. Potatoes are a whole food and are fine to eat when you bake them or boil them. Also if you haven't already figured it out, French people do not really eat French fries.

One problem with French fries is that they are usually deep friend in trans fats. As we have discussed, these saturated fats are very bad and have been linked to heart disease, diabetes and cancer. These bad fats also clog arteries. The same applies with French fries. French fries also have high levels of Acrylamide, which has been shown to possibly cause cancer. Dr. Mercola, one of the experts that Frank is a big fan of regularly tells people "One French fry is worse for your health than one cigarette."

Bacon

Plenty of people put bacon among their favorite foods. A strip of bacon has about 40 calories and 4 grams of fat with about 1.5-2 grams coming from saturated fat. However, this is another food you should never eat again. Bacon is high in salt and also in nitrates. It also has most of its calories coming from fat.

Nitrates are preservatives that are used in many processed foods. They can also be found in hot dogs and sausage. One of the reasons that nitrates are so bad for you is that they have been linked to cancer. In an article called "Meaty Diet May Raise Pancreatic Cancer Risk," WebMD news mentions that, "nitrite-based meat preservation techniques may be responsible for the increase in pancreatic cancer risk." This article also recounted studies on the topic including one that said people who ate high levels of pork had a 50% higher risk of pancreatic cancer. It is believed that this illness results from the meat preparation techniques in processed meats.

Nitrates also may contribute to chronic obstructive pulmonary disease. A study recently published in the American Journal of Respiratory and Critical Care Medicine followed over 7000 people over 45 years old who eat cured meats like bacon versus those who did not. The results showed that people who eat 14 or more servings a month are more likely to develop chronic obstructive pulmonary disease. The researches in this study suspect that the nitrates and antimicrobial agents and color fixatives may be responsible for this damage.

Who would have thought that bacon could be bad for your lungs as well as your waistline? This fact just serves to exemplify the dangers of processed foods. If you must eat bacon, just make sure it is nitrate-free.

Non-Dairy Products

Countless people put a non-dairy creamer in their coffee every morning. They may even consume more than one creamer as they go throughout the day. Non-dairy creamers can be very convenient in areas where there is no refrigerator to keep some fresh cream or milk for coffee cold. People who enjoy the taste of cream in their coffee but are lactose intolerant also often choose nondairy creamers. However, non-dairy creamer and other non-dairy products are really toxic and should be eliminated from your diet for good.

So what is wrong with non-dairy products? For starters, they are often made up of transfats. They also commonly include corn syrup. The word is out—some non-dairy creamer companies get away with saying that there is "zero transfat." But that is only because the portion size is low for just one cup of coffee and can be considered about .5 grams of fat per serving. Food companies are allowed to round this low number down to zero. Of course, when you start to use more than one teaspoon or non-dairy creamer in multiple cups of coffee, the level of trans fat that you are consuming will really make a difference to your health.

Similar to non-dairy creamer, non-dairy topping (often put on ice cream or jello) has partially hydrogenated oils and corn syrup. Preservatives are also usually added into the mix as well. These non-dairy creamer toppings may be used on desserts that you aren't even aware of. Some places even use it to top off hot chocolate.

If you can handle dairy, some low-fat milk or even a touch of half and half is better for your good health. If you are trying to avoid dairy, opt for soy creamer or rice milk.

Frozen Dinners

When people need a fast meal and know they won't have time to cook, it is easy to stock up on frozen dinners. While there are some organic frozen dinner selections that are ok to eat, most frozen dinners are fully processed. These frozen meals are also frequently stripped of the nutrients that would normally be in food. Frozen dinners can be a likely place for transfats, artificial flavors, artificial colorings, chemicals, preservatives and high levels of sugar and salt.

Another harmful element that is often found in frozen dinners is high fructose corn syrup. It is found items that vary widely, from frozen dinners, to breads to soft drinks and ketchup. High fructose corn syrup is bad for us for a variety of reasons. It depletes the body of chromium; it also is believed to encourage overeating. High fructose corn syrup also is often called "corn sweetener" or "corn syrup."

Men's Health magazine recently wrote an article June 2009 called "the Best Worst and Best! Microwave Meals." This article has some interesting facts about the dangers of frozen dinners. For example, Stouffer's Bourbon Steak Tips have a large amount of transfat with "oil" showing up three times in the ingredients. Also there is 1120 mg of sodium in this dinner than can be very harmful for people, especially those with high blood pressure. If you are opting for pizza, some frozen dinners likewise are very bad for the body. For example, Di Giorno For One Traditional Crust Pepperoni has 770 calories and again, an off the chart level of trans fat. Even though the pizza says it is for one, it has enough calories and fat to feed two or three people.

Incidentally, if you are looking for good frozen foods, there is one company that we recommend and that is Amy's Kitchen. Every now and then, of course, you won't have time to prepare a healthy meal, and you will want something fast and easy. Amy's meals are completely organic. In fact, Amy's Kitchen was producing healthy organic frozen meals before most people knew what the word "organic" meant. Amy's kitchen offers a wide variety of organic and non-GMO foods including pizzas, burritos, and desserts. Amy's Kitchen has recently gotten tons of commendations from Health Magazine, Reader's Digest and Los Angeles Daily News.

Movie Theater Popcorn and Microwave Popcorn

The Center for Science in the Public Interest recently wrote an article about movie theatre popcorn entitled "Two Thumbs Down for Movie Theatre Popcorn." This article includes a variety of interesting details about popcorn amongst which is that medium popcorn and soda combo at the popular movie chain Regal, has 1,610 calories 60 grams of saturated fat. The amount of fat is normal for 3 days. AMC and Cinemark's popcorn also have obscenely high levels of calories and fat. The AMC large popcorn has 1030 calories and 57 grams of fat. Cinemark's large popcorn has 910 calories and 4 grams of fat due to the heart healthy canola oil they use. Yes, Cinemark's popcorn has far less fat.

However, don't run to Cinemark for a popcorn just yet. This popcorn at Cinemark has 1500 milligrams of sodium, which is double the sodium in Regal or AMC's popcorn. The Center for Science in the Public Interest writes, "a large popcorn without topping from Cinemark will be less likely to clog your arteries but more likely to elevate your blood pressure."

But going home and using microwave popcorn may make things even worse. Some experts are now espousing the dangers of microwave popcorn. An FDA report recently showed that a chemical that coats the inside of microwave popcorn bag breaks down into a potentially carcinogenic substance called perfluorooctanoic. Also diacetyl has been found in microwave popcorn's fake butter.

Currently, there are a variety of lawsuits on "popcorn worker's lung." This is an illness experienced by people who worked in factories, which make microwave popcorn, who got too much exposure to the diacetyl fumes. Also people who eat a lot of microwave popcorns have had illnesses that have been attributd to diacetyl. This includes people with lung caner and even a few deaths. AOL news, WebMD, and The Wall Street Journal have both recently covered stories on the dangers of microwave popcorn.

So whether you choose popcorn from the movies or at home in your microwave, you are potentially facing dangers. What is the solution? You can pop popcorn on your stove the old fashioned way. Look for our popcorn recipe in the recipe section of this book.

Chapter 15
HOW TO EAT RIGHT

"We begin to see, therefore, the importance of selecting our environment with the greatest of care, because environment is the mental feeding ground out of which the food that goes into our minds is extracted." —Napoleon Hill

Be Your Own Cheerleader-Seriously

One of the first steps that you must take towards eating right is to be your own cheerleader. You shouldn't be depending upon outside influences for your inspiration and motivation in terms of achieving your fitness goals. The bottom line is that you need to remember that your attitude is key to your success. It is your determination and belief in yourself that will guide you towards your goals.

If you need help or have an off day, that is fine. After all, you are human. But try and alter your mindset, if necessary, to that of being your own cheerleader.

Be Your Own Friend

"Being your own friend" and dropping a few pounds might not seem like they are linked. Many people go through life beating themselves up for their own lack of success. Ask yourself what good such behavior is and what it accomplishes. This type of behavior will not lead to any tangible results in your goal of eating right.

... think long and hard about how you are going to approach your fitness goals.

Eating right, dropping pounds and achieving your fitness goals isn't completely about will power. There is a very real element of strategy as well. It is necessary for you to roll up your sleeves and think long and hard about how you are going to approach your fitness goals.

The Twelve First Steps Towards Eating Right

1. Step one may sound silly, but it's truly the foundation of all that will follow. You must want to change your diet. If you don't want to change your diet and instead you want to keep eating the way you have always eaten, then your goals will be difficult to reach indeed.

2. Remove your negative thinking from your mind. True, this is easier said that done, but its very important to embrace this step if you are going to meet your fitness goals and eat a healthier diet.

3. Access those around you who may be influencing how you eat and behave. If you have people in your life that may be influencing how you behave towards food, you may have to either stop associating with them or address this point. Perhaps it may be as simple as stating to them what your dietary and fitness goals are. This may be enough to help them see that they need to help and support you in this regard.

4. Avoid the places that might interfere with your diet if possible. This is not to state that you must avoid going to the grocery store. However, that doesn't mean that you should linger in the cookie or ice cream section either. But although you do have to go to the grocery store for food, you do not have to go to fast food restaurants.

   Fast food restaurants are simply dangerous places for those looking to eat healthy food and live a healthy lifestyle. You can read plenty of books that will tell you that if you select "this" or "that" off of a given menu you will be "okay," but this is sort of ridiculous. Studies have shown that often calories and fat are often not even listed accurately by fast food restaurants. Plus, there is the issue of temptation. Why risk it?

5. Try and find a "nutrition buddy." A nutrition buddy is someone who will share your goals and attempt to keep you on track. If you have a friend that you know is a healthier eater than you currently are, then ask them for help. Its okay to ask people for help, you just shouldn't depend on that help for your ultimate success. Remember you should be your own cheerleader and your own friend; you should believe in your nutrition and fitness goals first and foremost.

6. If you have friends who are eating healthier and have been doing so for years, then ask them for help. Don't be shy to "pick their brains" and find out what strategies they use to eat healthier.

7. Set aside more time to shop the healthy way. The reason that this point is important is that you will need to spend more time learning about food. You will also need to spend more time at the grocery store examining what is and is not a healthy option. Set aside some time in your schedule to relearn how to shop.

8. Also set aside time to read books on health and nutrition. It is not necessary that you spend an hour a day reading on health and nutrition. Even five minutes is enough. If you don't have five minutes, well, your stress level is way to high and you need to address that immediately! Here is the reason that this point is important. Reading and learning about health and nutrition is one thing that you can do to keep your mind focused on being healthy and sticking to your nutrition plan. Remember, like attracts like. The more you are focusing your mind on healthy information, the more likely you are to become healthy and achieve your goals.

9. Always remember the importance of hydration. Drinking plenty of water is a major first step. Most people are rarely properly hydrated and this is very important in terms of being healthy. Moreover, proper hydration will mean that you eat less as well. So it's a good idea to start focusing on your water intake even before launching a new way of eating.

10. Don't push too hard, too fast. Trying to cut your calories in half, for example, is really the kind dietary decision that must be made with a doctor and under medical supervision. The bottom line is that you are not dieting; you are working to adopt a healthy lifestyle and eat better, higher quality food. If you push to hard and don't give your body time to adapt your will power will be tested.

11. Consult your doctor about your plan. It makes good sense to get a physical if you have not had one recently anyway. See what additional advice your doctor may have in terms of adopting your new, healthier lifestyle as well.

12. Have a good time. If you are reading those words, "have a good time" and thinking "yeah right," then you are approaching the concept of adopting a healthier way of eating all wrong. You are changing your diet; you are not giving up food. With a little patience, work and experimentation, you will find hosts of new ways to prepare food, new foods to eat and new strategies for enjoying food.

This should be seen as the beginning of a new culinary journey and not a funeral for food your "old long-lost friend." Eating is fun, and there is no reason you can't still have fun. In fact, you must enjoy your food if you are to be successful over the long haul.

The Law of Attraction and Eating Right

The Law of Attraction can most certainly be used to help you improve the overall quality of your diet. Just imagine for a moment that you begin to eat all high-quality fruits, vegetables, grains and nuts, for example. The more you give these quality foods to your body, the more your body will crave them. Your biology will literally attract more of the same, and in this case it's something very good, into your life.

By taking that first positive step towards improving your own health, the universe will work to reward you with ever improving health. Your body will begin to crave the nutrition of these foods because you will simply feel better when you are eating them.

The Law of Attraction and Eating Poorly

Consequently, if you are eating foods that are full of chemicals, unhealthy fats and preservatives, then your body will crave more of those unhealthy elements. In a sense you can see the Law of Attraction at work here in a rather straightforward and easy to understand way. Like attracts like. If you are eating healthy food you will want more healthy food. If you are eating unhealthy food, then you will want more unhealthy food.

Talk to anyone that has ever switched over from an unhealthy diet to a healthy diet and you will usually find out that they begin to crave the healthier foods after a few weeks. After a few months, they usually have a very strong craving for these healthy foods.

Now this is not to state that you will not have cravings for the foods you once ate on a less than healthy diet, as you might very well have these cravings too. However, you will find that most of the time your body will begin to crave healthier choices. Part of the trick is to give your body the opportunity to say, "I like this… more of this please." This is the Law of Attraction at work and this is how you can use the Law of Attraction to help you fulfill your goal of eating a healthier and more life giving diet. It's not impossible; it is just a matter of proper strategy and approach.

Making The Change

Change can sometimes be tricky and difficult. Having the right approach to change is thus very important. When you set out to completely change your diet make sure that you have a workable and sensible plan. You shouldn't expect that you would completely transform your diet in the first day or the first week. The truth is that a complete dietary transformation will take most people a certain degree of time. Focus on introducing various healthy foods into your diet, and try and not get discouraged.

Getting discouraged can be a major factor for those who are dieting, and this is a key point that you need to remember. You are not dieting. Bringing all these healthy foods into your diet is not about the short term; instead, it is about the long term. You should use this book to help guide your dietary choices. Part of how you can do this is by consulting the various recipes at the end of this book. And when you are done reading our healthy recipes, go out and buy some healthy cookbooks and learn yet more recipes that sound intriguing. Eating should be fun, and you should work to make sure that your new dietary habits are making you happy.

The Law of Attraction and Believing You Can Do It

The Law of Attraction dictates that if you are happy with what you are eating, you will continue to eat in this fashion. This leads to another important point. One must also exercise a degree of patience. You should not expect your body to instantly stop craving the unhealthy food you are accustomed to eating. Consider that this is the food your body is used to eating, and it is only natural that you will crave this food for a period.

But be patient. If you began working out after years of being very inactive, you wouldn't start out the first day expecting to be able to bench press 300 pounds or run a marathon. If you told people that these were your expectations, they would quite seriously believe you were insane.

You should treat your new healthy eating habits in a similar fashion. By respecting the process and realizing that it will naturally take some time, you will dramatically increase your odds of success. The term dramatically can't be overemphasized in regards to this essential point. Be patient, be confident, be focused and you will achieve your goal of a becoming a healthier eater!

The Mediterranean Diet

We are big proponents of the Mediterranean Diet. This is a cooking style that very much reflects the eating habits of those living in the countries on the Mediterranean Sea. This diet is believed to lower the risk of heart attacks substantially.

The Mediterranean Diet is very much in tune with the Law of Attraction. It does not emphasize restriction and what you cannot have. Instead, this diet focuses on eating and enjoying the most fresh and healthy foods that are available. The meals do not end up seeming restrictive, but instead they turn out to be satisfying and delicious.

The Mediterranean Diet stresses:

1. **A diet rich in fresh fruits, vegetables, nuts and grains.**

   People in the Mediterranean usually eat very little meat. They eat lots of fruits and vegetables, along with rice. It is always best to eat foods in season that are also local. When you import fruit and vegetable from the other side of the planet, not only is it bad for the environment, the produce also loses some of its nutritional value during transit.

2. **A Diet with healthy fats**

   Most foods are whole foods in The Mediterranean Diet. There is little exposure to trans fats. In fact, there is a great deal of extra virgin olive oil in this diet. (That, of course, you would expect being that everyone associates olives with Greece.) Extra virgin olive oil is the type of oil that is least processed. Therefore, you still get the protective plant compounds with extra virgin olive oil. Nuts also provide healthy fats including linolenic acid, which is an omega3 fatty acid.

3. **Red wine**

   The Mediterranean Diet includes red wine. Red wine is associated with the anti-aging compound resveratrol. It also contains antioxidants. Don't go crazy with the wine, however. Experts at the Mayo clinic suggest no more than 5 oz of red wine a day for women and no more than 10 oz a day of wine for men under 65. According to the Mayo clinic, wine over this amount can potentially cause health problems including cancer. Do feel free to drink red wine, but take it easy.

4. **Seafood**

   Those living in the Mediterranean eat lots of fish due to their location on the sea. We recommend eating seafood once or twice a week. Always avoid fried fish though. It is best to grill or bake the fish.

5. **Attention to portion size**

   The Mediterranean Diet stresses small portion sizes. You can feel totally satisfied and full when you eat only a small amount of high quality food. This is a much better option than gorging yourself on food that has less nutritional value. You will also stay full longer because you are satisfying your body with the healthy, nutritious foods it requires.

Supplements

Another part of a healthy diet is to start incorporating supplements into your diet. Even when we are trying to eat the best diet, it is not always possible to get all of the nutrients that our body needs. Unfortunately, in modern day society, we are often too busy or distracted to find the time to get our body exactly the right nutrients day after day. This is a goal you should strive for, but it is difficult to achieve total perfection.

Obviously, there is an extremely wide range of supplements out there. It can be a bit overwhelming to even know which ones are actually necessary. Here are our recommendations for the supplements you should be looking at to achieve optimum health.

Whole Food Supplements

If you feel as though your diet is lacking in any way, shape or form, it is a good idea to take a whole food supplement. These vitamins originate from actual food sources as opposed to chemical compounds. How do you know if you are dealing with a whole food supplement? Take a look at the back of the bottle and see if the ingredients say that they are derived from actual natural sources. If so, you will see fruits and vegetables listed instead of just chemical names.

Whole food supplements also frequently contain organic herbs and antioxidants. In addition to your typical rundown of essential vitamins and minerals, in whole food supplements, you can find a wide variety of beneficial added ingredients like shitake mushroom and dandelion. All of these ingredients work in a synergistic manner to improve your overall health.

Omega 3 Supplements

Omega 3 is a fatty acid that is essential for the body, but omegas are only available in a limited amount of foods. You can mainly find them in seafood (salmon, sardines, mackerel) and some nuts. If you don't typically eat seafood and nuts, you may be lacking in omega 3. We recommend taking over the counter fish oil to get more omega 3 into your diet. However, make sure that you are taking a high quality fish oil to avoid accidental exposure to pollutants and mercury.

Conjugated Linoleic Acid

Conjugated Linoleic Acid or CLA is a unique fatty acid with some extremely beneficial properties. In studies, CLA has been shown to stop cancer, increase the immune system, reduce inflammation, and balance blood sugar. It has also been shown to have positive effects on high cholesterol and blood pressure.

Apparently, conjugated linoleic acid can also help with weight loss. Here is some information about CLA from the book *The Natural Fat-Loss Pharmacy: Drug-Free Remedies to Help You Safely Lose Weight* by Harry Preuss and Bill Gottlieb. "In research conducted in Japan, America, Canada, Australia and Poland, curious scientists conducted experiments on the body fat of various species of laboratory animals, feeding some a CLA-enriched diet, while others didn't get CLA. In most of those studies, the CLA animals ended up with much less body fat and much more lean body mass than animals not fed CLA."

Another interesting thing that has been showed in studies of people taking CLA, is that people on it didn't gain back their fat years later. As a result, it is highly recommended for maintaining weight loss results. A supplement that is great for the body and also helps to achieve and maintain a healthy weight is definitely something worth looking into.

Alpha Lipoic Acid

Alpha Lipoic acid is produced in the body naturally and also acts as an antioxidant. It can also neutralize free radicals in the body and prevent them from damaging cells. Some foods do contain alpha lipoic acid naturally, including spinach, liver, yams, broccoli, tomatos, carrots and brewer's yeast. In *The Healing Power of Vitamins, Minerals, and Herbs* By Reader's Digest, the writer's state, "Its difficult, however, to obtain therapeutic amounts of this vitaminlike substance through diet alone. Instead, many experts recommend using supplements to get the full benefits of alpha lipoid acid." When you take alpha lipoic acid as a supplement, the body's tissues easily absorb it.

In the book *Alpha Lipoic Acid: Nature's Ultimate Antioxidant*

By Allen Sosin, Beth Ley Jacobs, the authors write, "In recent years a new generation of antioxidants have hit the supplement shelves, and the best and brightest of them is Alpha Lipoic Acid. This versatile antioxidant has the unique ability to neutralize both water and fat-soluble free radicals as well as rejuvenate other antioxidants back into their active, protective forms. Alpha Lipoic Acid is also essential for energy production and the metabolism of sugar."

Alpha lipoic acid can treat the conditions of people with diabetes because its antioxidants can counteract damage to the nerves. It also can protect the liver against poisons or toxic chemicals. Alpha lipoic acid has also been shown to boost the immune system. It has also been shown to remove mercury from the body.

Resveratrol

Resveratrol is a compound that is believed by scientists to contribute to longevity. Studies have also shown it may protect against cancer and help those with diabetes. Resvertrol occurs naturally in red wine, Spanish peanuts, whole grape skins, raspberries and mulberries. In a landmark study, fruit flies and worms were shown to have significantly longer lives when they were given resveratrol.

Initially resveratrol was studied as part of what is called the "French Paradox." The paradox is that French people are less likely to have heart disease and tend to live longer, healthier lives. Yet, French people smoke cigarettes and eat foods high in fat. On the other hand, the French drink lots of red wine.

In a 2007 issue of Fortune Magazine entitled "Can Red Wine Help You Live Forever?" David Stipp writes about resveratrol. "Resveratrol is the ingredient in red wine that made headlines in November when scientists demonstrated that it kept overfed mice from gaining weight, turned them into the equivalent of Olympic marathoners, and seemed to slow down their aging process. Few medical discoveries have generated so much instant buzz." However, studies on resveratrol are still in their early stages.

Although there is currently pills coming from Sirtris Pharmaceuticals, health expert Dr. Mercola recommends waiting until this company has established more a reputation before taking their resveratrol based drugs. Instead he recommends getting more natural sources of resveratrol like whole grape skins, raspberries and mulberries.

White Tea

White tea is something that is easy to incorporate into your diet. Like green tea, white tea has been used as medicine for centuries. However, white tea is perhaps even more essential because it is the least processed form of tea. It also has the highest levels of antioxidants. This tea is picked before the tea buds have a chance to open.

Antioxidants, of course, prevent damage to the body by way of free radicals. Antioxidants like those in white tea can neutralize these free radicals. White tea also has flavonoids. Flavonoids are a type of antioxidant that is shown to fight cancer cells. If you can reduce your risk of cancer just by drinking tea, why not go for it?

Also white tea have a host of other health benefits which include lowering blood pressure and cholesterol, protecting your heart and making your bones stronger. It is also antibacterial and antiviral. This means it can protect you against diseases and even the common cold.

White tea also has an amino acid called theanine. This compound is believed to have mood enhancing properties. The amount of caffeine in white tea is fairly low, so you don't have to worry so much about caffeine withdrawal or the tea interfering with your ability to sleep unless you are unusually sensitive.

Chapter 16
BENEFITS OF HEALTHY LIVING

"Nothing will benefit human health and increase chances for survival of life on Earth as much as the evolution to a vegetarian diet." —Albert Einstein

How Healthy Living Will Benefit You

Many people fail to appreciate just how much they can be helped from proper nutrition and exercise. There is a notion that many have that being healthy might slightly improve their lives, but that the overall impact really won't be that great. Nothing could be further from the truth.

In this chapter, you will see that being healthy through proper diet and exercise can work wonders and can greatly improve your life in a variety of ways. This chapter should help you get motivated not just to get into shape and start eating healthy for a short period of time, but also to keep doing so for the rest of your life.

The bottom line is that being healthy will give you an edge in life. It will help you accomplish what you are looking to accomplish. By combining a healthy lifestyle with the Law of Attraction, you will be taking advance of a powerful combination. These two elements may see like they are very far apart, but the truth of the matter is that a healthy diet, exercise and the Law of Attraction are linked in a variety of ways.

We all want to be happy. Being healthy is a way to accomplish the goal of being happy. While some of the ways this works may not be initially obvious, they are nonetheless effective. The benefits of healthy living are most definitely not limited to simply having a lower blood pressure score or being able to run a mile in a given number of minutes. Instead the ways that healthy living can impact your life radiate out in various directions.

When you add up all the different ways that healthy living can make your life better, you will become addicted to the idea. You will wonder why you haven't been living a healthy lifestyle all along. Some of the reasons that your life will improve can be explained on a very practical level. Other ways that your life will improve are not quite possible to explain tangibly because they are the result of the Law of Attraction working on your behalf to achieve your greatest desires.

In this chapter, we will explore exactly how you will benefit from a healthy lifestyle and how it can and will impact your life on a personal and professional level. Whatever it is that you are seeking more of in your life, a healthy lifestyle can quickly help you receive in a more expedient fashion. Using the Law of Attraction and healthy living together will produce serious and long lasting chance in your life.

Healthy Living and Personal and Professional Success

We all want to have happy personal lives and happy professional lives. Of course, what we define as happiness and what we might quantify as success will no doubt vary. No matter what your definition of personal and professional success might be, being healthy will help you achieve those goals.

Here are a few ways that adopting a healthy lifestyle can help you achieve your goals.

Ten Ways That A Healthy Lifestyle Can Help You Achieve Your Goals

1.   You have probably heard that attitude is everything. And to some extent this statement is hard to deny. A positive attitude is the launching point for any successful endeavor, whether personal or professional. Belief is key in all endeavors.

     If you believe you can do something, then there is a chance of success. Obviously if you don't believe something is possible, then you are instantly correct. A healthy person is much more likely to be able to have a positive outlook than an unhealthy person.

2.   If you feel horrible due to illness, then the odds are you will not be able to roll up your sleeves and accomplish great things. Just think back to the last time you had a cold or flu. Odds are that you didn't feel too motivated.

     When your body is fighting of an infection, cold or flu, you don't feel much like doing anything. This is where being healthy and embracing a healthy lifestyle come into play. If you feel miserable, you will not be able to tackle your goals. The first step towards staying healthy is your diet and your level of exercise.

3. Diet and exercise will impact your immune system. There are powerful chemicals found in foods, such as fruits and vegetables, which work to make your immune system stronger. By lacking healthy foods in your diet, you are forcing your immune system to work more and you will get sick more often. This translates into less time feeling well and less time accomplishing your goals.

4. Adopting a healthy lifestyle will save you money over the long term. Eating healthy foods and taking time to workout may seem at first as though it is costing you money. But the fact of the matter is that this is preventative medicine and an investment in you! While you may spend more on food by adopting a healthy lifestyle, you will be spending less money in other areas.

    For example, a person with a healthy lifestyle will be drinking very little, if any, alcohol, will not be smoking and will skip spending money on expensive, high-calorie coffee drinks. By spending that money on healthy food, instead you will also be avoiding many of the diseases associated with drinking and smoking.

    The impact of substances such as alcohol and tobacco can have serious health consequences and even cause death. If you are sick with an illness, you will obviously be losing money. You can't accomplish your goals if you are dead either! Thus, prevention is key.

5. A healthy person will save on doctor's bills. Doctor's bills are expensive, and this is especially evident when those bills greatly exceed what a insurance company covers. People across the country are quite literally going bankrupt everyday due to medical bills. By embracing a healthy lifestyle, many medical problems can be delayed for years, decades or even eliminated altogether. And how do we put a price on suffering? A healthy person will not have to suffer from illness.

6. You can probably remember in your own life a time when you were ill and ended up feeling depressed. Depressed people clearly have trouble accomplishing their goals. By staying healthy, you will avoid the depression that is often associated with sickness. Clearly, avoiding depression is important. After all, the core of achieving your goals is to maintain an optimistic attitude and feel positive energy. Numerous medical studies have shown that there is a link between food and mood. This can be especially true if you are eating foods you are allergic to and do not even realize it.

7. A healthy lifestyle will, in all likelihood, mean that you live longer. A good many people enjoy dismissing this fact with the extraordinarily absurd line of logic that goes along the lines of "I could get hit by a train tomorrow so why bother." Why bother getting out of bed or brushing your teeth then? This primitive line of logic is widely practiced and is not a type of thinking

that someone who accomplishes his or her goals will take. If you want to succeed, you should avoid this type of "logic" at all cost!

8. Living longer increases you chances of having a happier life, especially if you embrace a healthy lifestyle. By living longer, you will have more chances to find happiness in your life and accomplish your goals. It's that simple.

   For example, you may indeed live long enough to see your grandchildren get married or play with your great grandchildren. Modern medical science in the last decade has taken tremendous leaps forward, and we will soon be witnessing an entire new array of medical breakthroughs and medical possibilities hit the market.

   Diseases that killed our parents and grandparents may soon be a thing of the past. Live long enough to see this happen and you might indeed be playing with your great grandchildren and maybe even doing so in decent health. That is serious personal happiness.

9. Have you ever had a fight with a friend or spouse because you felt poorly? The odds are that you have. When we are sick, we are quite literally not ourselves. As a result, we will get into fights that would otherwise have been totally avoided or will seem completely foolish when we are in better health. If you are living a healthy lifestyle, you will be feeling better. If you are feeling better you will have more personal happiness in your life. This fact should radiate out to all of your personal relationships and relationships in general.

10. If you are happy and healthy, you are more likely to reach out and attempt things that you would have otherwise maybe not imagined. In a sense, living your life as a consistently healthy person will change who you are. You will spend more time working toward your goals and doing what makes you happy. Now how can you argue with that?

Striving to be happy and being physically healthy are indeed linked in ways that many people fail to see. It is important that you see the benefits of being healthy and embrace them into your own life. There is no doubt that the Law of Attraction works and that you can attract and draw into your own life what you desire and need.

It is important that you see the benefits of being healthy and embrace them into your own life.

Excitingly, there is a way that you can make the Law of Attraction work even better for you. By simply eating healthy foods and getting a little exercise, you will give your body and mind more energy, and you will feel better. At the end of the day, you will have accomplished more.

Healthy Living Plus the Law of Attraction Can Give You A Professional and Business Edge

You have likely heard that the Law of Attraction can give you an edge in your professional life, but healthy living can serve as a serious way to boost the effectiveness of the Law of Attraction in this regard. There are a variety of ways that a healthy lifestyle can be incorporated into the Law of Attraction in order to make achieving your overall professional goals more likely.

Just as we have established that a healthy lifestyle through proper nutrition and exercise can help one achieve their goals, the same can be said for business. The logic behind this couldn't be much simpler.

Imagine there are two women, Samantha and Jenny. Lets say that both are about equally skilled at the same jobs, but Samantha frequently gets sick and takes time off from work. Just based upon that fact, which of these two women do you think is more likely to get a promotion? This greatly underscores how being healthy gives one a real and substantial edge professionally.

Don't Overlook The Healthy Living Edge

It is nothing short of amazing how people will consistently look for all sorts of edges in business, yet often overlook some of the most basic ones possible, such as staying healthy. Many people are resistant to change and do not want to give up what they have become accustomed to in life, whether that if a particular kind of food or alcohol or a variety of other unhealthy habits. But this is exactly how using a healthy lifestyle together with the Law of Attraction can help you.

A healthy lifestyle will make you feel better, and this will radiate out in all sorts of ways that will help you reach your professional and business goals. The trick is to not be afraid to embrace these changes.

Don't Be Afraid To Strike Out On Your Own

Sadly, many people will fail to embrace the changes necessary in their lives out of fear of what others will think. Peer pressure can be powerful at any age. Often people will not adopt heavy lifestyle choices because those around them are not encouraging or helpful. It may be necessary to ignore what others have to say in regards to your health goals. You know that living a healthy lifestyle is linked to your achieving of your overall goals. This may mean ignoring any negative input you get from those around you.

Remember that to use the Law of Attraction effectively, you need to focus on what you want and to do so intensely. If you have people in your life who do not understand your healthy lifestyle choices, then it's okay to ignore them or in some cases distance yourself from them. Don't be afraid to strike out on your own!

Ten Ways That A Healthy Lifestyle Will Help Your Professional and Business Goals

1. In business, having a positive outlook is definitely important. No matter what your profession (or even if you are an entrepreneur), being positive will undoubtedly yield results. Let's think about Samantha and Jenny again. Let's say that both women are equally skilled at accounting. However, Jenny is wildly more positive than Samantha. Again, who is mostly likely to get ahead?

    While many variables are involved, most of the time, most people would agree that Jenny would get ahead. Usually, in most settings, the person that is upbeat and easy to get along with will go further in a company or business. Employers will appreciate the good attitude as they realize that attitude can be infectious. Other employees will like having Jenny around and, in turn, the office environment will run smoother.

2. The person with a positive outlook on life is more likely to see ways of solving problems. Which person is more likely to see a novel way to solve a problem or address a situation, the person that is depressed or the person that is positive and upbeat? This is why a healthy diet and a healthy lifestyle are so critical in achieving one's professional goals. The person with the healthy lifestyle is more likely to feel good and remain healthy year round. That could very well turn out to be a significant edge over the long haul!

3. By living a healthy lifestyle, one is more likely to stay healthy. If you are healthy, you are able to work toward your goals. Also this means that if you are healthy, you are able to not just show up for work with greater frequency. You will also able to perform better when you are at work.

    Employers notice factors such as a sick employee. They also notice employees that never seem to get sick and are always on the job. Come time for an important promotion to a critical position, there is little doubt that such a factor is considered carefully before the final hiring decision is reached. In a close competition for a job, this detail could make all the difference!

4. Employers and customers also notice energy levels. Energy level denotes a great many things. For example, it should how much someone is enjoying their job and it says a great deal about their attitude as well. Employers also realize that attitude can be contagious and factor this is as well.

    A sluggish person is one that seems as though he or she doesn't care too much. Whether or not the sluggish employee does care may be irrelevant as the perception is that he or she does not care. For this reason, the person with the higher energy level has a clear edge. He will be more likely to make that sale or accomplish that goal.

    Likewise, entrepreneurs need tremendous amounts of energy, and thus, this principle applies to them as well. If you are working for yourself, you want to have the best energy and stamina to get a lot of work done in a shorter period of time. The energy and enthusiasm you have can directly result in money in the bank! Yet, if you are working for yourself and get sick, the converse is true. Each day that you aren't working can make a huge difference in your earnings and the success of your business. In short, a healthy lifestyle will mean more energy and that will translate into a better job performance and a better perception of you as well!

5. There is little doubt that a healthy lifestyle will mean better stamina. You won't just be able to be energetic for part of the day; instead, you will be a consistent performer day in and day again. Again, being able to work throughout the day is critical for an entrepreneur as well. This is yet another way that a healthy lifestyle can give you the edge.

6. By adopting a healthy diet, you are making sure that you avoid the highs and lows that are often associated with sugary snacks, such as the donut or several teaspoons of sugar in the morning coffee. Eating healthy food throughout the day helps insure that you will not have the post-lunch lag or experience similar food related issues. This will increase your productivity. It all comes courtesy of having a healthy diet.

7. Eating more nutritious healthy food both on the job and after hours will no doubt improve your mood. Just as avoiding the highs and lows of the sugar rush will help you be more productive, it will also help you regulate your mood.

    Being moody at work is just a bad idea, whether you are working in an office or operating heavy machinery. Anything that you can do to ensure that you do not have mood swings is extremely beneficial. Eliminating those, "I wish I had no said that moments," is enough to justify eating a healthy diet all on its own!

8. While we would all like to pretend that we do not live in a "looks-based" superficial society, who are we kidding? Clearly, looks matter a great deal.

Most people are impacted by looks at a subconscious level at the very least. If you look unhealthy, it could impact how coworkers, employers or potential clients perceive you.

Looking healthy and fit is a definite way to give you an edge in the business world. A healthy diet and a healthy lifestyle can be great help in this regard. It would be nice to think that the most qualified and hardest working person always gets the job, but this is just not always the case. It can actually help you to achieve your goals by looking younger and having a healthy glow.

9. If you adopt a healthy lifestyle, you are far less likely to spend time at the doctor's office. An occasion trip to the doctor or sick day isn't likely to be seen as too much of a blemish on most people's work records. However, if too many afternoon visits to the doctor start piling up, a negative perception might be the end result. Eating healthy foods and getting enough exercise can go a very long way in reducing illness in general.

10. Longevity is an important aspect of achieving all of your goals in life. If you are dead, well, you are dead. That is pretty much it for you and your goals in life. A healthy lifestyle will make sure that you stay alive longer, and that can impact your goals in a variety of ways.

The Many, Varied Benefits of Healthy Living

At this point, the various benefits of having a healthy lifestyle should be very obvious. Combining smart food choices, exercise and the Law of Attraction will help you reach your personal and professional goals. For some people, diet and exercise might seem like a way to get a "small" edge in life, but when one steps back and considers all the ways that a healthy lifestyle can help one achieve one's goals, the end result is staggering.

Simply adopting a healthy diet can go a long way in reducing a wide variety of sicknesses and illnesses that might take you out of commission. Not being able to strive to reach your goals can impact your overall attitude.

It should be obvious from this chapter that everything is interlinked. You may have noticed how many of the various points where somehow linked to one another and this is no mistake. Your performance is linked to how you feel and this is linked to your attitude and perceptions. This, of course, underscores how important a healthy lifestyle is for success. If a good attitude is critical to success, then just consider how important a healthy lifestyle is for success.

If you truly want to reach your goals, then you will strive to make sure that you are as healthy as possible. Don't you want to be the best you that you can possibly be? By not optimizing your health, you are not being the best person that you can be.

Thinking carefully about how you spend your food dollars and how you treat your food decisions could very well turn out to be critical in your overall success. Many people waste large sums of money on food and drink items that they do not need, but are also harming their health and even causing disease in the process. For those who want to be both successful and healthy, this makes no sense. Success and health are most definitely linked.

Determination and Eating Right

Many people decide that they are going to eat a healthier and more nutritious diet. But the real challenge is to make sure that we stick with a plan. Most of us have made New Year's Resolutions that we are going to start exercising or start eating right. Unfortunately, most people find it difficult to stick to these resolutions and goals.

Saying to yourself, "I am going to start eating right, I am going to start eating healthy," is a big part of the challenge. Yet, another aspect of the challenge that is not quite so obvious is that you need to completely believe in your own success. You need to know down to your very core that you are going to start eating in a totally different way.

You need to see your goal as not being to eat better for a while but permanently. In this regard, you may have to permanently change the way that you see and approach food. Remember that one of your goals is to shed your extra pounds and say good-bye to them for good. There is no reason that you should feel as though accomplishing this goal is impossible. People are successfully accomplishing their fitness and health goals everyday and you can too.

Part Three

HEALTHY RECIPES

Chapter 17

INTRODUCTION TO RECIPES

The last part of this book includes a variety of healthy recipes for you to choose from. These are some of our healthy favorites, and they are recipes that are specifically designed to be nutritious, flavorful and easy to prepare.

There are clearly a seemingly endless amount of food choices. The number of food choices in fact skyrocket when one incorporates items such as processed foods into the mix. Part of reaching one's goal of having a healthier diet is to zero in on what foods should be avoided.

When choosing your own recipes, here are some types of foods that should be avoided. We already covered some of this information in the 10 Superfoods and 10 Foods You Should Never Eat Again chapters.

Recap of What to Avoid

Here is a quick recap of foods to avoid. These are all foods that will not only pack on the pounds, but they will also deplete your energy level. Unhealthy foods can make you feel stressed, tired, and depleted of energy. When you want the Law of Attraction to work on your behalf, follow these guidelines.

1. Skip processed foods. The more you can avoid processed foods the better. All of the recipes that you choose should be made out of whole foods.

2. Avoid fast food. Don't think of fast food as a food that you can have once a day, as you should just try to forget that it even exists!

3. Fattening foods full of unhealthy fats should not be on the table. Luckily most of those foods, but not all, are processed foods. Avoid trans fats such as the increasingly famous partially hydrogenated oils. Consuming too much

of these unhealthy fats can lead to a variety of diseases, including heart disease. In a word, you don't need this stuff. You will see in our recipes only include healthy oils such as extra virgin olive oil and coconut oil.

4.   Soft drinks should probably be removed from your list of foods that you can eat. Stating that you can't give up soft drinks is the same thing as stating that you can't stand the idea of changing your diet. Soft drinks are complete empty calories, with no nutritional value at all and are loaded down with sugar and chemicals. If tough love needs to be applied anywhere in this book it is probably on the point of soft drinks. And forget about the diet soft drinks. Eating healthy means getting the chemicals out of your diet and diet soft drinks are not magic; they are chemicals.

5.   You will need to become an avid label reader. Look at labels whenever you get a chance and find those chemicals. Part of getting eating right and eating healthy is to dump the chemicals and preservatives. Just like trans fats, you don't need chemicals in your diet.

6.   Meats, poultry, eggs and dairy that are non-organic should be taken off your table if you want to have a healthy diet. Unfortunately non-organic meats, poultry, eggs and diary have some serious issues such as the animals being given growth hormones and massive doses of antibiotics. If possible, choose free-range and grass fed options when available. When you are making the recipes in this book, try to opt for as much organic food as possible. However, when you do opt for these foods, just be sure to always go organic.

7.   Farm raised fish is a food that you should skip. Testing consistently shows that farm raised fish, such as farm-raised salmon has a variety of contaminants. We have a section of recipes on wild Alaskan salmon recipes. Just make sure that your salmon is always wild Alaskan.

8.   A little red wine is fine here and there, but you definitely want to go easy on alcohol. Yes, I know you had an aunt or cousin that lived to be ninety-three and they were a raging alcoholic, but that doesn't mean you will live to be ninety-three. Alcohol, for the most part, is empty calories and that means you should just skip it.

9.   If you are eating white bread, pasta or white flour you should definitely switch to a healthier alternative. There is far more nutrition in whole-wheat pasta and whole wheat breads for example. White flour products are really just poor imitations of real grain products.

10.   Number ten on our list of foods you should avoid is seriously important; foods that make you feel bad. So many of us have stopped listening to our bodies and that is very, very bad. If a food is making you feel badly then why eat it. Also it's important to factor in how a food makes you feel an hour or two after you have eaten.

The sugar rush of sweets, for example, is a great example. You might feel good while eating it, but even a few minutes later this is probably going to be a different story. Keep this important point in mind and let your body guide you to better food choices. If you learn to listen you can be guided to make better choices through how you feel.

The Best Foods

Our recipes that you are about to read are just a sampling of how you can create delicious meals with the healthiest ingredients. And its not just our recipes, we encourage you to start exploring new healthy recipes on the Internet and in books. There is a world of extremely healthy, life-supporting foods and new recipes that you may not even know about. Once you get started, these foods will very likely become some of your new favorites.

Here is a quick overview of some of the food principles that are incorporated into our recipes.

1. By now you have heard that vegetables are good for you. It is often strange to hear people say that they don't like vegetables, considering that there are so many different kinds of vegetables in the world. Experimenting, no matter what the subject may be, will broaden your horizons and serve to make you a more interesting person. So experiment with different vegetables until you find ones that you like. Eating vegetables with lots of rich, vibrant color is a great place to start. Make sure you find ways to incorporate green leafy vegetables as well.

2. Learn to eat salads if you do not already do so. Once again, experiment and find salad dressings and vegetables that you like. A good salad will be full of vitamins and minerals that your body is craving. Eating one salad a day will dramatically improve your health, especially over the long term.

3. Yes, where vegetables are discussed, fruits are soon to follow. Fruits and vegetables do make for a great nutritional combination when one is looking to improve the diet. Just as vegetables are loaded down with nutrients, the same can be stated concerning fruits. Here is another big point to remember. Fruits and vegetables are loaded down with antioxidants, which will keep your body from aging.

4. Feel free to go a little nuts. Most of us get the major majority of our protein from animal sources, but there are some amazing protein sources that were never walking or swimming around. Walnuts, for example, are loaded with omega-3 fatty acids that are simply fantastic for your brain and your heart and they are also anti-inflammatory. Toss a few walnuts into that salad every

day or consider adding other nuts. Nuts are a great way to get lots of protein, vitamins and minerals without eating animal protein.

5.　The egg has been given a rough ride in recent years due to the cholesterol levels. A little cholesterol is necessary in the human body. The problem was that so many people had high cholesterol levels from other foods that they were eating that the last thing they needed was more cholesterol. Yet the egg is an amazing source of protein and has very few calories. Now isn't that exactly the kind of protein that anyone looking to shed a few pounds should be interested in?

6.　Find a place for fish on your table. The reason that you may have heard about the importance of eating fish in the media in recent years is due to the omega-3 fatty acids contained in fish. Fish is a great way to get your protein and your omega-3 fatty acids at the same time. When choosing fish two of the very best are wild Alaskan salmon and sardines, as both are high in omega-3 fatty acids.

Salmon should be wild Alaskan and not farm raised, however. Here is one additional important point to keep in mind. All fish contains contaminates such as mercury, yes mercury, and other heavy metals. One has to keep this in mind when selecting fish. For this reason, fish like tuna, which is high in mercury, should usually be avoided. This is especially true for pregnant women.

7.　So far we have covered that you should be eating vegetables, fruits, salads, nuts, eggs and quality seafood (such as wild Alaskans salmon and sardines). But these are obviously not the only foods you should eat. Yet, it is definitely a good start. Introducing as many of these foods into your diet as possible is a sure fire way to see pounds drop and your health improve.

While it is true that fruits, vegetables and nuts all have fiber, there is a food that you should be eating all the time due to its high fiber and protein levels. That food is beans. Often people think that beans are too simple to be a major contributor to an overall healthy diet, but nothing could be further from the truth. Beans are a true winner as they are packed with vitamins, minerals, protein and fiber.

8.　Extra virgin olive oil has been proven to be a true nutritional winner. Extra virgin olive oil is full of healthy fats, but is also been shown to prevent numerous diseases. In fact, one could argue that olive oil is among the healthiest of all foods you can eat.

9.　Yogurt and kefir should be on your list if you consume dairy. The probiotics found in both kefir and yogurt will help you keep your digestive system in good working order. For those of you who do not eat diary, consider coconut kefir or soy yogurt as a replacement.

10. Consult your superfoods list found in this book. The superfoods list in this book is full of many can't miss foods that will improve your diet. They are commonly available foods that are sure to make a big impact on your overall health.

Some Background Information about Our Recommendations

We just wanted to add a few additional notes that will assist you as you go through the recipes section.

- In many of the recipes, salt is incorporated. When we indicate, "Salt," we want to point out that we are always recommending crystal salt. Not only does a crystal salt like Himalayan crystal salt taste better, it is also healthier for you. Regular table salt has been stripped of its minerals. However, the remaining salt is over processed and not healthy for the body.

- You will notice in our pasta recipes, we opt for brown rice pasta. As the name indicates, brown rice pasta is made from brown rice. This means that it is gluten-free, trans-fat free, cholesterol free and wheat-free. One brand in particular that we recommend is Tinkyada. Regular pasta is high on the glycemic index. This means that it the glucose in the food is released rapidly into your bloodstream. Researchers believe that foods high on the glycemic index increase the risk of obesity. In general, pasta is not a very healthy food.

  However, the pasta that really needs to be avoided is that which is made from wheat. It is high in calories and has little nutritional benefit. Sure, if you go to restaurants and order pasta every now and then, it is ok. However, regular pasta is not a staple that you should eat at home if you want to achieve and maintain optimum health. The best pasta to eat is brown rice pasta. If you cannot obtain brown rice pasta, whole-wheat pasta or spelt pasta would be the next best choice.

- We have recommended sardines in this book. However, not all sardines are the same level of quality. A company that consistently produces high quality sardines is Vital Choice. These sardines are high in omega 3 and low in sodium. They are also packed in organic extra virgin olive oil. This company also sells high quality salmon, and eco-fish.

- When you are going through our recipes, please keep in mind that all the ingredients should be organic. Organic foods are always going to be the best for your body since they are free of chemicals and pesticides. Please incorporate as much organic food as you can when you prepare your meals.

Kale Recipes

We are going to start our recipes with 3 delicious kale recipes. Kale typically isn't a vegetable that most people opt for. However, if you properly prepare kale, it can be extremely tasty. Once you have begun acclimating your tastebuds to healthier foods, kale will very likely be one of the vegetables that you crave! Yes, this may be hard to believe right now if you are not a fan of kale. However, stick with this vegetable and give it a chance. The rewards will likely be very gratifying.

Easy Raw Kale Recipe

Serves 2-3

Most people think that raw kale seems as though a method of preparation that would be impossible to enjoy. The trick is to massage the kale by hand instead of just stirring or tossing it. When you mix salt and lemon into kale by hand, the fibrous chewy element of the kale breaks down to something soft and quite delicious.

Ingredients

1 kale
3 cloves of garlic
1 lemon
1-tablespoon tahini
1-teaspoon extra virgin olive oil
1 tablespoon of sesame seeds or hemp seeds
Salt
Pepper
Cayenne Pepper

Directions

1. Chop the kale into very small pieces (the smaller, the better)

2. Put kale in a bowl and add garlic, tahini, olive oil, 1-teaspoon salt, 1-teaspoon pepper, 1-teaspoon cayenne pepper, and the juice of one lemon.

3. Put your hands into the bowl and massage the kale thoroughly. Make sure each part of the kale is massaged. The lemon and salt helps to break down the kale.

4. Let marinate for 5-10 minutes.

5. Top with sesame or hemp seeds.

6. Serve.

Kale Chips

Believe it or not, kale makes a great substitution for potato chips. This simple recipe is great to have on hand the next time you feel as though you want a chip. However, keep in mind how much better you will feel on the inside and outside when you know your chip is made out of kale.

Ingredients

1 kale
Salt
Extra virgin olive oil

Directions

1. Preheat oven to 350 F.

2. Tear kale into pieces the size of chips. You do not need to worry about removing the stems.

3. Spread kale on a cookie sheet.

4. Put your extra virgin olive oil in a spray bottle and spray the kale lightly. If you do not have a spray bottle, you can lightly rub a minimal amount of oil into each kale chip.

5. Sprinkle kale with salt.

6. Bake for about 10 minutes. The kale should be crispy when you are done.

Kale with Almonds

Serves 2

This easy kale dish makes stars out of two extremely healthy ingredients: kale and almonds. If you avoid soy, you can also substitute Bragg's liquid aminos. If you only have peanut butter, you can also use it instead of the almond butter. (Peanut butter is a lot less expensive and also works well in this dish.)

Ingredients

Brown rice
1 kale
½ onion
2 garlic cloves

Extra virgin olive oil
½ teaspoon coriander
¼ teaspoon chili powder
2 tablespoons tamari
¼ cup almond butter
1 cup chopped almonds
Salt
Pepper

Directions

1. Chop onion and garlic.

2. In a bowl, mix almond butter, tamari, ¼ cup filtered water, spices and 1-teaspoon salt.

3. Blend the spices into this sauce thoroughly.

4. Heat 1-tablespoon olive oil.

5. Sauté onion and garlic in pan.

6. Add kale to pan and cook until wilted.

7. Add the almond sauce and stir to coat kale.

8. Serve on plate with brown rice.

9. Top with chopped almonds.

10. Season with salt and pepper to taste.

Blueberry Recipes

We have discussed blueberries earlier in the book in the Superfoods chapter. Blueberries may be small, but these little guys are much tougher than they look and much more nutritious as well. A serving of blueberries contains powerful phytonutrients called anthocyanidins. These anthocyanidins, work to fight oxidative damage in one's body. Foods high in antioxidants like blueberries can help your body deal with all the oxidative stress that it is under. Oxidative stress is what causes your body to break down and any food rich in antioxidants, like blueberries, helps fight this process.

Blueberries are rather high in antioxidants and other compounds that help fight off scores of diseases, including many cancers. Blueberries can been found to help fight inflammation in the body as well. Meaning that this little blue wonders can help you recover fast from an injury.

Delicious Breakfast Oatmeal

Serves 2-3

Steel cut oats are healthier than other oats like quick oats because they are less processed and, as a result, have more nutritional content. Whole oats have soluble fiber, selenium, thiamine, phosphorus, and manganese

Ingredients

1-cup steel cut oats
½ cup raisins
1-cup blueberries (preferably fresh blueberries, frozen ones are also ok)
Agave nectar
Cinnamon

Directions

1. Add 1 cup steel oats to pot.

2. Add two cups of filtered water, stir, and bring to boil.

3. Add ½ cup raisins to the pot.

4. Cook for about 20 minutes, stirring occasionally.

5. Take off heat and divide into bowls.

6. Top each bowl with blueberries.

7. Sprinkle 1-teaspoon cinnamon on each bowl of oatmeal.

8. Drizzle 1 teaspoon of agave on each bowl.

Top with any or all of the following (or use any healthy ingredient you can imagine. It is time to get creative.)

Milks: Soymilk, almond milk, walnut milk…
Nuts: Almonds, walnuts, sunflower seeds, flax seeds, pecans…
Fruit: Pineapple, Banana, apple, fresh cherries, peaches, pumpkin puree…
Dried fruit: Cranberries, dried cherries, dates, apricots, etc…

Oatmeal Muffins with Blueberries

Makes 12 Muffins

These muffins make a great healthy dessert or breakfast. They are also fantastic on the go. They have a slightly granola-like flavor. If you want a slightly less sweet muffin, you can also make these without the agave.

Ingredients

½ cup applesauce
¼ cup agave
3 cups oats
2 eggs
1 cup almond milk or soymilk
1-tablespoon baking powder
½ teaspoon salt
1-teaspoon cinnamon
½ cup raisins
½ cup blueberries

Directions

1. Preheat over to 350F.
2. Combine all ingredients into large bowl.
3. Mix well.
4. Get a muffin or cupcake pan and grease the pan with olive oil or coconut oil.
5. Fill each cupcake with batter.
6. Bake for 25 minutes.

Blueberry Smoothie #1

This smoothie is a great idea for something to turn to when you are craving a dessert like ice cream. This smoothie has a very satisfying cold and icy consistency. It also will totally satisfy your sweet tooth. If you don't have bananas, you can also substitute strawberries and the smoothie will be just as good. Also if you are looking for a slightly less sweet smoothie, just leave out the agave.

Ingredients

1 large frozen banana
½ cup almond milk or soymilk
1-cup yoghurt or kefir
1 teaspoon flax seed
1-teaspoon agave
2/3 cup frozen blueberries

Directions

1. Cut banana into chunks.

2. Add nut milk, yoghurt, flax seed, and agave.

3. Blend on low speed.

4. While the speed is still low, slowly add blueberries.

5. Once blueberries are blended, turn blender on high.

6. Blend for a minute more and then pour into glasses.

Orange Blueberry Smoothie

This is a truly refreshing drink that is great anytime of year. Frozen blueberries will also work if you can't find fresh blueberries. You can also alternate strawberries and raspberries into this recipe.

Ingredients

1 ripe banana
¼ cup almond milk or soymilk
¼ cup orange juice
½ teaspoon vanilla
¼ cup yoghurt or kefir
1-teaspoon agave
1-cup blueberries

Directions

1. Combine nut milk and bananas in blender.

2. Blend until smooth.

3. Add orange juice, vanilla, yoghurt, and agave.

4. Blend on low.

5. Add blueberries.

6. Continue to blend on low.

Summary

These are just the first 6 of our favorite recipes for healthy foods. Instead of breaking the recipes down into categories like breakfast, snacks and dinners, these recipes are arranged by ingredient. Each chapter highlights a particular superfood as the star of the menu.

Chapter 18

TOMATO RECIPES

Tomatoes have a variety of health benefits. One of the best reasons to eat tomatoes is for the lycopene. Lycopene is a powerful antioxidant that fights against cancer cells. It also protects the body against other diseases as well. The tomato has by far the highest concentration of lycopene than any other fruit or vegetable. If you are looking for the most lycopene in your tomatoes, always choose ones that are organic.

Channa Masala

Serves 4

Channa Masala is a delicious Indian dish that is moderately easy to make. The great thing about most Indian dishes is that you get a lot of bang for your buck in the way of spices. It is also fantastic to get turmeric into any meal that you can fit it into.

Ingredients

1 can of chickpeas
1-Tablespoon Ghee or coconut oil
1 onion
2 garlic cloves
1 Lemon
2 cups cherry tomatoes
1-Tablespoon Coriander
1-Teaspoon Cumin
1-Teaspoon Turmeric
1 Teaspoon garam masala
1-cup basmati rice

Jalapeno pepper
Fresh Ginger
Salt
Pepper
Cayenne Pepper

Directions

1. Chop ½ jalapeno, onions and garlic.

2. Dice cherry tomatoes.

3. Grate 2 teaspoons ginger.

4. Heat pan (with lid) to medium and add ghee.

5. Sautee onions and garlic until tender.

6. Add all spices except garam masala and cook for about 15 seconds stirring well to blend spices in with onions and garlic.

7. Stir in tomatoes and cook for about 5 minutes.

8. Bring chickpeas and 1 cup water to boil.

9. Once mixture has boiled, put lid on pan and turn it down to simmer for 10 minutes.

10. Add garam masala, jalapeno and juice of a lemon. Put lid back on for 5 minutes.

11. Season with salt, pepper and cayenne pepper to taste.

12. Serve with basmati rice.

Recipe Checklist for Channa Masala

- Skill Level Required-Low (While there are a dozen steps, this one is reasonably easy.)

- Ease of Preparation Grade-B+

- Speed of Preparation Grade-B

- Protein Grade-C

- Low Calorie-Yes

- Number of Nutritional Superstars-12 (Chickpeas, onion, cloves, lemon, tomatoes, coriander, cumin, turmeric, garam masala, jalapeño pepper, ginger, cayenne pepper.)

- Raw, Cooked or Both-Cooked

- Good For Entertaining-Yes

Recipe Wrap-Up

This dish should be a hit with guests and your own taste buds at the same time. If you find yourself craving foods and want something different, a dish like Channa Masala should help reduce your cravings a bit.

Vegan Tomato Soup

Serves 4

This tomato soup may sound boring, but it has a great deal of complexity of flavor and a very gourmet feel.

Ingredients

2 shallots
½ onion
3 garlic cloves
Jalapeno pepper
Coconut oil
30 oz can tomato sauce
15 oz can diced tomatoes
2 tomatoes
½ cup coconut milk
½ cup white wine
1 bunch fresh basil
Salt
Pepper
Cayenne Pepper

Directions

1. Chop ½ jalapeno, onions, shallots and garlic.

2. Sautee jalapeno, onions, shallots and garlic in coconut oil until onions and shallots are transparent.

3. Add wine and cook on medium heat for 2-3 minutes.

4. Chop 2 tomatoes and chop basil.

5. Add into pot tomato sauce, tomatoes, diced tomatoes, coconut milk, basil, and ½ cup water.

6. Serve with seasonings of salt, pepper and cayenne pepper.

Recipe Checklist for Vegan Tomato Soup

- Skill Level Required-Low
- Ease of Preparation Grade-A
- Speed of Preparation Grade-A
- Protein Grade-C-
- Low Calorie-Yes
- Number of Nutritional Superstars-9 (Shallots, onions, garlic, Jalapeno peppers, coconut oil, tomatoes, coconut milk and cayenne pepper.)
- Raw, Cooked or Both-Cooked
- Good For Entertaining-Yes

Recipe Wrap-Up

Recipes don't come too much easier than the Vegan Tomato Soup recipe. Now this is not to state that this recipe isn't quite good. In fact, you might be pretty surprised with the overall results. People might just tell you that it's the tastiest tomato soup they've ever had!

Vegetable and Cashew Soup

Serves 4

This vegetable cashew soup is a great variation on the typical tomato soup flavors. The drizzle of cashew cream at the end of the recipe also gives it an exotic look and taste.

Ingredients

2 shallots
1 small onion
4 garlic cloves
Coconut oil
1-cup raw cashews
1-cup almond milk or soymilk
4 carrots
6 plum tomatoes
1 bay leaf
1 15 oz can tomato paste
Salt
Pepper

Directions

1. Place raw cashews in a small bowl and cover with filtered water. Let the cashews soak for at least 5 hours, preferably overnight.

2. Drain cashews and put in the blender with 1 cup of milk.

3. Set aside cashew mixture.

4. Chop shallots, onion and garlic cloves.

5. Dice carrots and cut tomatoes into small pieces.

6. Heat a pot and add 1 Tablespoon coconut oil.

7. Sauce shallots, onion and garlic cloves until onion and garlic are translucent.

8. Add carrots, tomatoes and bay leaf to the pot.

9. Add three cups of filtered water.

10. Simmer for 45 minutes.

11. Remove bay leaf.

12. Add tomato paste to the pot.

13. Use blender or food processor to blend soup.

14. Pour soup back in pot.

15. Ladle soup into bowls.

16. Drizzle each bowl of soup with cashew mixture.

17. Season with salt and pepper and serve.

Recipe Checklist for Vegetable and Cashew Soup

- Skill Level Required-Medium
- Ease of Preparation Grade-C+
- Speed of Preparation Grade-C-
- Protein Grade-B
- Low Calorie-Yes
- Number of Nutritional Superstars-10
- Raw, Cooked or Both-Cooked
- Good For Entertaining-Maybe

Recipe Wrap-Up

Whether or not you wish to tackle this recipe for entertaining depends largely on your schedule and level of comfort in the kitchen. This is a very tasty recipe, but the Vegetable and Cashew Soup does take some preparation time.

Tabbouleh

Serves 4

Tabbouleh is a Middle Eastern dish that typically accompanies meat dishes. However, tabbouleh makes a great meal and can hold its own. If you make hummus, this is a great dish to compliment your meal.

Ingredients

½ cup bulgar wheat
1 lemon
Extra virgin olive oil
3 cloves of garlic
1 stalk of green onion
¾ cup fresh parsley
¼ cup fresh cilantro
¼ cup fresh mint
1 cucumber
2 cups plum tomato
Salt
Pepper
Cayenne Pepper

Directions:

1. Boil ¾ cup water.

2. Add bulgar wheat to pot.

3. Take off heat and let stand 20 minutes.

4. Chop green onions, parsely, cilantro and mint.

5. Dice garlic.

6. Dice cucumber and tomato.

7. Add the bulgar wheat, green onions, parsley, cilantro, mint, garlic, cucumber and tomato together in a bowl.

8.   Add 1-2 tablespoons extra virgin olive oil.

9.   Squeeze one lemon into bowl.

10. Add salt, pepper and cayenne pepper to taste.

11. Stir well.

12. Refrigerate for an hour before serving.

Recipe Checklist for Tabbouleh
- Skill Level Required-Low
- Ease of Preparation Grade-A-
- Speed of Preparation Grade-B
- Protein Grade-C
- Low Calorie-Yes
- Number of Nutritional Superstars-11
- Raw, Cooked or Both-Both
- Good For Entertaining-Yes

Recipe Wrap-Up

This is a filling low calorie meal that dieters will learn to love and appreciate. Considering that tabbouleh is even better the second day, this is one recipe you are probably going to love.

Gazpacho

Serves 4-5

Gazpacho is a summertime favorite that is also very healthy. This is also a perfect soup to cure you if you are ever sick in the summer. Gazpacho also goes over really well for entertaining. It's a soup that most people like, but they don't often get a chance to have.

Ingredients

1 lemon
Extra virgin olive oil
3 cloves of garlic
1 stalk of green onion

¾ cup fresh parsley
¼ cup fresh cilantro
¼ cup fresh basil
1 cucumber
8 plum tomatoes
2 shallots
3 tablespoons balsamic vinegar
1 green pepper
1-teaspoon agave
Salt
Pepper
Cayenne Pepper

Directions

1. Add to blender the following: juice of one lemon, 2 tablespoons extra virgin olive oil, 1 green onion, 1 cucumber, tomatoes, shallots, 3 tablespoons balsamic vinegar, green pepper, 1 teaspoon cayenne pepper and agave.

2. Blend until smooth.

3. Serve in bowls and season with salt and pepper to taste.

Recipe Checklist for Gazpacho

- Skill Level Required-Low
- Ease of Preparation Grade-A
- Speed of Preparation Grade-A
- Protein Grade-C
- Low Calorie-Yes
- Number of Nutritional Superstars-11 (Olive oil, garlic, onion, parsley, cilantro, basil, cucumber, tomatoes, shallots, green pepper and cayenne pepper.)
- Raw, Cooked or Both-Raw
- Good For Entertaining-Yes

Recipe Wrap-Up

If you want to look sophisticated but don't have much time to prepare a dinner for guests, consider the mighty gazpacho. Also if you are looking for easy to prepare meals that are raw and vegan, this will become one of your go-to recipes.

Healthy Vegetarian Chili

Serves 4

This chili recipe is very easy to make. One great thing about it is that if you keep your pantry stocked with beans and tomatoes, this is a great recipe for times that you are running out of food and haven't yet had time to go shopping. Healthy vegetarian chili is more satisfying and filling than just ordering a pizza.

Ingredients

One large onion
5 cloves garlic
1 15-ounce can of diced tomatoes
1 28-ounce can of crushed tomatoes
4 tomatoes
1 green pepper
1 red pepper
1 15-ounce can of kidney beans
1 15-ounce can of pinto beans
Chili Powder
Salt
Pepper
Cayenne Pepper
1-tablespoon oregano

Directions

1. Dice onion and garlic.
2. Dice green pepper, red pepper and tomatoes.
3. Add 1 tablespoon of olive oil to pot.
4. Add onions and garlic.
5. Cook until onions are translucent.
6. Add the following items to the pot: peppers, tomatoes, both cans of tomatoes, kidney beans, pinto beans, 2 teaspoons of chili powder, 1 teaspoon of salt and 1 teaspoon of pepper.
7. Bring to boil.
8. Reduce heat and simmer for 15 minutes.
9. Stir in one tablespoon of oregano.
10. Season with salt, pepper and cayenne pepper as necessary.

Recipe Checklist for Healthy Vegetarian Chili

- Skill Level Required-Low
- Ease of Preparation Grade-A-
- Speed of Preparation Grade-B+
- Protein Grade-A-
- Low Calorie-Yes
- Number of Nutritional Superstars-11
- Raw, Cooked or Both-Cooked
- Good For Entertaining-Yes

Recipe Wrap-Up

Healthy Vegetarian Chili is a must for dieters and for good reason. Since this recipe has two kinds of beans, you can be sure that it has a good deal of protein, fiber, vitamins and minerals. If you are particularly hungry, then you simply can't go wrong with this wonderful recipe.

Chapter 19

BLACK BEAN RECIPES

Black beans are a great addition to your diet for a variety of reasons. They have a great deal of dietary fiber. Black beans are also high in antioxidants and fight free radicals that can lead to disease and aging. Black beans also have higher levels of flavonoids than other beans. Another major plus for black beans is that they have been shown to lower cholesterol levels and reduce heart attack risks. When you combine black beans with a whole grain or brown rice, you get a similar protein makeup to a food like dairy or meat.

Quinoa Stuffed Peppers

Serves 4

When you eat these quinoa stuffed peppers, you won't miss the meat at all. The mushrooms and black beans serve as a tasty substitution.

Ingredients

Extra virgin olive oil
1 onion
4 cloves of garlic
2 cups Portobello mushrooms
Cayenne pepper
Cumin
1 15 oz can tomato sauce
1 can black beans
½ cup quinoa
2 large green peppers
2 large red peppers
Salt

Directions

1. Preheat the oven to 350 Fahrenheit.
2. Chop onions and mushrooms into small pieces.
3. Mince garlic.
4. Add 2 tablespoons olive oil to pot.
5. Add onions and sauté for a few minutes until soft.
6. Add garlic and mushrooms and sauté for another 3-5 minutes.
7. Stir in 1-teaspoon cayenne pepper, 1-teaspoon cumin, and 1-teaspoon salt.
8. Add quinoa and ¼ cup water. Simmer for 15 minutes.
9. After 15 minutes, take mixture off of heat and stir in 1 cup of tomato sauce and black beans.
10. Cut the top off of each pepper and throw away seeds.
11. Boil a large pot of water.
12. Once water is boiling, drop whole peppers into the water for 3-5 minutes.
13. Place each pepper on baking dish with the interior pointing upwards.
14. Fill each pepper with mushroom mixture.
15. Cover the top of each pepper with tomato sauce.
16. Bake for 20 minutes.

Recipe Checklist for Quinoa Stuffed Peppers

- Skill Level Required-Medium
- Ease of Preparation Grade-C
- Speed of Preparation Grade-C
- Protein Grade-B
- Low Calorie-Yes
- Number of Nutritional Superstars-11
- Raw, Cooked or Both-Cooked
- Good For Entertaining-Yes

Recipe Wrap-Up

The fact that this dish has mushrooms and quinoa gives it some extra protein. Most people think that this dish is substantially more difficult than it is to make. If you serve quinoa stuffed peppers for guests, they will think that you have prepared something quite elaborate.

Vegan Black Bean Soup

Serves 4

This vegan black bean soup recipe is very hearty and filling. If you can tolerate lots of spice, feel free to throw in lots of cayenne and oregano. You can also consider topping the soup with some organic hot sauce for an added kick. Another variation on the soup is to add additional vegetables. When you add in the corn, you can also add in red or green peppers, celery, or diced carrots.

This is a very low calorie soup. If you want to add in some healthy fat, serve each bowl of soup with a slice of avocado.

Ingredients

Extra Virgin Olive Oil
1 onion
4 cloves of garlic
3 carrots
1 ½ Tablespoons chili powder
1-tablespoon cumin
4 cups vegetable broth
2 cans black beans
1 15 oz can diced tomatoes
1 12 oz bag frozen corn
1 green onion
Salt
Pepper
Cayenne pepper
Oregano
Avocado (optional)

Directions

1. Dice onion and carrots.

2. Mince 3 cloves of garlic.

3. Heat 1 Tablespoon of olive oil over medium heat. Sauce onion, carrot and garlic for 3 minutes.

4. Add chili powder and cumin. Cook for 30 seconds.

5. Stir in vegetable broth and 1 can of beans and bring to a boil.

6. In the blender or food processor blend 1 can of beans, diced tomatoes, and one clove of garlic.

7. Add the contents of the blender to soup pot.

8. Add frozen corn to pot.

9. Simmer for 10 minutes.

10. Garnish with green onion slices.

11. Season with salt, pepper, cayenne pepper and oregano.

Recipe Checklist for Vegan Black Bean Soup

- Skill Level Required-Low

- Ease of Preparation Grade-B+

- Speed of Preparation Grade-B+

- Protein Grade-B

- Low Calorie-A

- Number of Nutritional Superstars-11 (Olive oil, onions, garlic, carrots, chili powder, cumin, black beans, tomatoes, cayenne pepper, oregano, avocado)

- Raw, Cooked or Both-Cooked

- Good For Entertaining-Yes

Recipe Wrap-Up

As far as soups are concerned, the Vegan Black Bean Soup is almost as easy as they come. Further, this soup is great for vegan, vegetarians and entertaining. This hearty soup is also great served with a slice of avocado.

Black Bean Veggie Burgers

Serves 2

This recipe serves as a great alternative to hamburgers and hotdogs. Instead of meat, you will be filling your body with high fiber beans, and lots of vegetables and spices. Although the instructions below take you through the process of baking the burgers, you can also feel free to put them right on the grill if you want to get the "outdoor experience."

You can also pair this burger with a spelt bun. However, try to get used to eating this burger with no bun. You will be surprised how easy it is to get used to having a burger this way.

Ingredients

One 15 oz can of black beans
1 red bell pepper
1 small onion
2 cloves garlic
1 egg
1-tablespoon chili powder
1-tablespoon cumin
1-teaspoon oregano
1-teaspoon salt
½ cup breadcrumbs
Organic salsa

Directions:

1. Preheat oven to 375 F.
2. Put a light coating of oil on a baking sheet.
3. In a food processor, blend pepper, onion, garlic, salt, cumin, oregano and chili powder.
4. In separate bowl, mash black beans.
5. Stir egg into the beans.
6. Add vegetable mixture into beans.
7. Add breadcrumbs and stir well.
8. Mixture should hold together and be fairly sticky.
9. Divide the mixture into four patties.
10. Bake burgers for 10 minutes on one side.
11. Turn over and bake burgers for 10 minutes on the other side.
12. Serve over salsa.

Recipe Checklist for Black Bean Burgers

- Skill Level Required-Medium
- Ease of Preparation Grade-C

- Speed of Preparation Grade-C
- Protein Grade-B
- Low Calorie-A
- Number of Nutritional Superstars-(Only salt and breadcrumbs fail to make the list.)
- Raw, Cooked or Both-Cooked
- Good For Entertaining-Yes

Recipe Wrap-Up

The Black Bean Veggie Burger definitely serves as a good, low-calorie, low-fat alternative to regular beef burgers. If you are looking for ways to consume less animal protein, then you might want to consider this burger, as it will be very filling and nutritious.

It is also important to point out that the Black Bean Burger has a good deal of fiber as well. Overall, this is a great alternative for dieters and one that may very well find its way into your weekly routine.

Black Bean Salad

Serves 2

One great thing about this black bean salad recipe is that it is very easy to put together quickly. It also is easy to commit this recipe to memory for when you are craving something good, but don't have a lot of time.

Ingredients

15 oz can of black beans
2 cups cherry tomato
1 red onion
2 cloves garlic
1-cup cilantro
Pumpkin seeds
Extra virgin olive oil
1 Lemon
Salt
Pepper
Cayenne Pepper

Directions

1. Mince garlic and dice onion.

2. Slice cherry tomatoes into quarters.

3. Chop cilantro coarsely.

4. Add garlic and onion into bowl.

5. Add can of black beans, tomatoes, ½ cup pumpkin seeds, and 2 tablespoons extra virgin olive oil.

6. Add cilantro and squeeze one lemon into bowl.

7. Toss the black bean salad well to blend ingredients.

8. Season with salt, pepper and cayenne pepper.

Recipe Checklist for Black Bean Salad

- Skill Level Required-Low

- Ease of Preparation Grade-A

- Speed of Preparation Grade-A

- Protein Grade-B

- Low Calorie-Yes

- Number of Nutritional Superstars-9 (Only salt and pepper don't make the list as nutritional superstars.)

- Raw, Cooked or Both-Raw

- Good For Entertaining-Yes

Recipe Wrap-Up

The Black Bean Salad is an easy, quick salad that is also high in protein and fiber—thanks to the black beans. Additionally, there is enough spice in the dish to definitely keep your taste buds interested. More than likely, you will find yourself whipping this one up more than once.

Black Bean Hummus

Serves 2

This black bean hummus is a delicious alternative to regular hummus. (Regular hummus is also quite healthy by the way. Just substitute chickpeas for the black beans if you want to try the standard recipe.) Hummus is a great recipe to be familiar with. It is easy to make, healthy and can usually be made with the ingredients that you already have in your pantry and refrigerator.

Ingredients

3 cloves of garlic
15 oz can of black beans
2 tablespoons raw tahini
Lemon
1-teaspoon cumin
Salt
Pepper
1 teaspoon Parsley
1 teaspoon Cayenne Pepper
1 Red Bell Pepper
1 Green Bell Pepper
5 carrots

Directions

1. In food processor, place 3 cloves of garlic. Pulse the food processor to puree garlic.

2. Add the following ingredients into the food processor: black beans, tahini, cumin, cayenne pepper, parsley, salt and pepper.

3. Squeeze the juice of one lemon into blender.

4. Blend until smooth.

5. Chop red peppers and green peppers into slices.

6. Cut carrots into carrot sticks.

7. Serve raw vegetables with the black bean hummus.

Recipe Checklist for Black Bean Hummus

- Skill Level Required-Low

- Ease of Preparation Grade-A

- Speed of Preparation Grade-A

- Protein Grade-B+
- Low Calorie-Yes (But exercise caution not to use too much tahini, which is high in calories.)
- Number of Nutritional Superstars-10
- Raw, Cooked or Both-Yes
- Good For Entertaining-Yes

Recipe Wrap-Up

Tossing ingredients into a food processor is pretty fast and easy. This fact helps make the Black Bean Hummus recipe a good one for a busy day. It takes very little preparation time. The end result seems much more elaborate than it actually is, and that is always a good thing.

Simplest Black Bean Dish

Serves 2

This really is a simple black bean dish. It is especially fast to make if you already have some brown rice prepared.

Ingredients

Brown rice
Extra virgin olive oil
Onion
1 red bell pepper
1 yellow or orange bell pepper
4 cloves of garlic
1 can of black beans
2 tablespoons apple cider vinegar
½ cup fresh cilantro
¼ cup cashews
Oregano
Salt
Pepper
Cayenne Pepper

Directions

1. Prepare brown rice and set aside.
2. Chop peppers and onions into small pieces.

3. Heat 1 tablespoon of olive oil on medium heat.

4. Sauté onion and garlic until onions are translucent.

5. Add peppers and sauté 1-2 minutes longer.

6. Add black beans, 1-teaspoon cayenne, and vinegar.

7. Simmer for 5 minutes.

8. Stir in rice.

9. Chop ½ cup of cilantro and stir into mixture.

10. Stir in cashews.

11. Season with salt and pepper.

Recipe Checklist for Simplest Black Bean Dish

- Skill Level Required-Low

- Ease of Preparation Grade-A-

- Speed of Preparation Grade-A-

- Protein Grade-B

- Low Calorie-A

- Number of Nutritional Superstars-11

- Raw, Cooked or Both-Cook

- Good For Entertaining-Yes

Recipe Wrap-Up

The Simplest Black Bean Dish, while being simple, has a very big and rather complex taste. This is, in part, due to the addition of apple cider vinegar and cashews.

Chapter 20
THE AVOCADO

Avocados are loaded with nutrition and healthy fats. Many people are still under the impression that all fats are bad fats but this just isn't the case. Avocados are high in several b Vitamins, vitamin C, zinc and several other vitamins and minerals.

Avocado Salad

Serves 2-3

This healthy salad is a great all-raw recipe that has a lot of flavor. If you want to have some added protein, you can always add in nuts (like cashews or almonds) or some red beans or garbanzo beans.

Ingredients

3 cups diced tomatoes
2 cucumbers
1 avocado
1 ½ cups cilantro
Extra virgin olive oil
3 limes
1-cup endive
Salt
Pepper
Cayenne Pepper

Directions

1. Cut avocado into small pieces.
2. Put avocado in small bowl and squeeze one lime into bowl.

3. Add one-teaspoon salt and ½ teaspoon cayenne.

4. Stir and set aside.

5. Chop tomatoes, endive and cucumber into bite sized pieces.

6. Add avocado mixture in with other vegetables.

7. Squeeze the additional three limes into bowl.

8. Add 1-tablespoon extra virgin olive oil.

9. Gently stir salad.

10. Season with salt, pepper and cayenne pepper as needed and serve immediately.

Recipe Checklist for Avocado Salad
*   Skill Level Required-Low
*   Ease of Preparation Grade-A
*   Speed of Preparation Grade-A
*   Protein Grade-C
*   Low Calorie-Yes
*   Number of Nutritional Superstars-6 (Tomatoes, avocado, cilantro, olive oil, cayenne pepper, endive)
*   Raw, Cooked or Both-Raw
*   Good For Entertaining-Yes

Recipe Wrap-Up

This simple avocado salad is a very healthy and nutritious meal and is perfect for easy dinners after a long day.

Kale Avocado Salad

Serves 4

Most people think that they don't like raw kale. But the secret is to give the kale a little "massage." When you massage kale by hand, the lemon juice and salt works to break down the fibers. The result is kale that is soft, spicy and delicious.

Ingredients

1 avocado
1 kale
1-cup tomato (this works best with cherry or plum tomatoes)
Lemon
Extra virgin olive oil
1 sheet Nori
Sesame Seeds
2 cloves garlic
Salt
Pepper
Cayenne Pepper

Directions

1. Chop the kale into small pieces and discard the stem.

2. Chop the tomato and garlic.

3. Break the nori into small squares.

4. Add into bowl the following: Avocado, Kale, juice of one lemon, tomato, nori, 2 tablespoons sesame or hemp seeds, garlic, 1 teaspoon salt, one teaspoon pepper and one teaspoon cayenne pepper.

5. Wash your hands and insert them into bowl. Instead of stirring, gently massage the kale with the other ingredients. Make sure you give all the pieces of kale a gentle massage.

Recipe Checklist for Kale Avocado Salad

• Skill Level Required-Low

• Ease of Preparation Grade-A

• Speed of Preparation Grade-A

• Protein Grade-C+ (The addition of nori to this recipe helps boost the overall level of protein.)

• Low Calorie-Yes

- Number of Nutritional Superstars-10
- Raw, Cooked or Both-Raw
- Good For Entertaining-Yes (This recipe is meant to serve four, and it couldn't be much easier to prepare.)

Recipe Wrap-Up

Most people don't eat enough seaweed and that is a shame. Seaweed has been shown to have a wide-array of benefits. The Kale Avocado Salad is a great one due to the fact that it's easy to make and is loaded with great, healthy ingredients. Kale and avocado in a single recipe is a reason to make this one frequently.

Raw Avocado Soup

Serves 4

Many people aren't fans of cold soup, but this raw avocado soup is good enough to make you a convert. The best thing of all is that you can add and subtract herbs, spices and vegetables depending on what you have in your kitchen, and the soup still turns out great. You can also try adding more herbs like thyme, oregano and parsley.

Ingredients

2 avocados
Lime
1-cup mint
½ cup cilantro
½ cup basil
1 cucumber
2 shallots
5 tomatillos
4 tomatoes
1 green bell pepper
1 red bell pepper
Extra virgin olive oil
Salt
Pepper
Cayenne Pepper
1 cup orange juice
1 cup pumpkin seeds

Directions

1. Add the following ingredients to the blender: 1 cup orange juice, 1 tablespoon olive oil, 1 green pepper (remove seeds), 1 cucumber, 5 tomatillos, 2 tomatoes, ½ cup basil, ½ cup cilantro, 2 avocados and 1 cup mint.

2. Add juice of one lime.

3. Blend thoroughly.

4. Chop red pepper and remaining 2 tomatoes into small bite sized chunks.

5. Add tomatoes and red pepper evenly to the bottom of bowls.

6. Pour avocado soup over the vegetables in the bowl.

7. Season as needed with salt, pepper and cayenne pepper.

8. Garnish with pumpkin seeds.

Recipe Checklist for Raw Avocado Soup

- Skill Level Required-Low
- Ease of Preparation Grade-A
- Speed of Preparation Grade-A
- Protein Grade-C+
- Low Calorie-Yes
- Number of Nutritional Superstars-15
- Raw, Cooked or Both-Raw
- Good For Entertaining-Yes

Recipe Wrap-Up

This is an absolutely fantastic recipe for entertaining. It is easy, quick and likely to be very big hit.

Pasta with Avocados

Serves 4

This dish is similar to vegan pesto pasta. However, the healthy fat of avocado substitutes for the cheese and pinenuts.

Ingredients

1 avocado
Brown rice pasta
3 cloves garlic
1 Tablespoon extra virgin olive oil
1 bunch basil
1-cup cherry tomatoes
2 tablespoons lemon juice (preferably from a fresh lemon)
Salt
Pepper
Cayenne Pepper

Directions

1. In the food processor add the following ingredients: garlic, lemon, basil, 1 teaspoon salt, 1 tablespoon extra virgin olive oil, 1 teaspoon pepper and 1-teaspoon cayenne pepper.

2. Blend until smooth.

3. Prepare brown rice pasta according to directions.

4. Drain pasta

5. Add avocado to pasta and toss.

6. Chop cherry tomatoes into halves.

7. Add cherry tomatoes to pasta.

8. Combine with food processor mixture and toss to blend all ingredients.

Recipe Checklist for Pasta with Avocados

- Skill Level Required-Low

- Ease of Preparation Grade-A

- Speed of Preparation Grade-A

- Protein Grade-B-

- Low Calorie-Yes (But watch the portion size.)

- Number of Nutritional Superstars-7 (avocado, garlic, olive oil, basil, tomatoes, lemon, cayenne pepper.)
- Raw, Cooked or Both-Both
- Good For Entertaining-Yes

Recipe Wrap-Up

Like most of the avocado dishes in this chapter, the Pasta with Avocados recipe is a great one for entertaining. Dieters should appreciate the fact that this recipe is very filling and puts an interesting new spin on traditional pasta.

Healthy Avocado Smoothie

Serves 2

You would not think that avocado would work so well in a smoothie, but it is the perfect way to get some healthy fats and also have a delicious "dessert-like" shake. You can use other fruits and experiment for the avocado shake that suits you best. You can also try adding fresh mint. Fresh mint and avocado are a great match.

Ingredients

½ avocado
1 frozen banana
2 strawberries (frozen or fresh)
½ cup frozen peaches
¼ cup of almond or soymilk
Pinch of cinnamon
Pinch of nutmeg

Directions

1. Blend all ingredients in a blender.
2. Serve and enjoy.

Recipe Checklist for Healthy Avocado Smoothie

- Skill Level Required-Low
- Ease of Preparation Grade-A
- Speed of Preparation Grade-A
- Protein Grade-C+

- Low Calorie-Yes
- Number of Nutritional Superstars-7 (Every ingredient qualifies.)
- Raw, Cooked or Both-Raw
- Good For Entertaining-Yes

Recipe Wrap-Up

You simply can't go wrong with this very yummy avocado smoothie. Just remember this smoothie isn't low calorie if you are having three a day. However, one is certainly fine.

Avocado Sushi with Sesame

Serves 2-3

If you love sushi but have never tried making it at home, now is your opportunity. You can also feel free to add additional fillings to your sushi. Tofu, sprouts, red pepper, and slices of wild Alaskan salmon or sardines all make good fillings.

Ingredients

1 cup of sushi rice
1 avocado
½ cucumber
5 nori sheets
2 Tablespoons sesame seeds
Small bowl of dipping water
Salt
2 Tablespoons Rice Vinegar
Cayenne Pepper

Directions

1. Add one cup of rice to small pot.
2. Add two cups of filtered water.
3. Bring to a boil.
4. Reduce heat to low and simmer for 5 -10 minutes.
5. Let rice cool.
6. Add 2 tablespoons of rice vinegar.

7. Add 1-teaspoon salt, 1-teaspoon cayenne pepper and 2 Tablespoons sesame seeds.

8. Stir rice well.

9. Slice avocado and cucumber into thin slices.

10. Lay out one sheet of nori with the shorter side closest to your body.

11. In the lower ¼ quadrant of the nori sheet, spread about 2 inches of the rice horizontally.

12. Lay thin slices of avocado and cucumber on top of the rice.

13. Hold the veggies and rice with your fingers and begin rolling the sushi into a cylindrical roll.

14. When you get to the end of the roll, dip your fingertips lightly in the water and use the water to fasten the ends of the roll together.

15. Repeat directions for the other 4 nori sheets.

16. Using a sharp serrated knife, slice each roll into bite-sized pieces about ¾ inch thick.

Recipe Checklist for Avocado Sushi with Sesame
- Skill Level Required-Medium
- Ease of Preparation Grade-C+
- Speed of Preparation Grade-C
- Protein Grade-C+
- Low Calorie-Yes
- Number of Nutritional Superstars-5 (Avocado, nori, sesame seeds, cayenne pepper and cucumber.)
- Raw, Cooked or Both-Both
- Good For Entertaining-Maybe

Recipe Wrap-Up

It should be noted that this is really only a dish for those who have practiced their sushi making skills. Few things are sadder than poorly executed sushi. Keep this in mind if you are tackling this recipe for guests.

Chapter 21

WILD ALASKAN SALMON AND SARDINE RECIPES

Wild Alaskan salmon is essential for our diet because of the healthy fats that it provides. Wild Alaskan salmon is high in essential omega-3 fatty acids, which have been shown to improve heart health and brain function. It is very important to note that only wild Alaskan salmon should be on your plate, preferably not Atlantic and most definitely not farm raised salmon. Some day the contamination problem with farm raised salmon might be addressed, but for now stick with wild Alaskan salmon. Wild Alaskan salmon is also high in protein.

Miso Soup with Wild Alaskan Salmon

Serves 2-3

This miso soup has a variety of superfoods in it. The soup can also be changed depending on which type of miso paste you choose. You should be able to find the miso easily at any health food store. Some regular grocery stores also carry it.

Ingredients

1 onion
4 cloves garlic
1 Tablespoon ginger
¾ pound Wild Alaskan Salmon
3 cups broccoli
Organic miso
1 leek

1-cup shitake mushrooms
1-tablespoon wakame seaweed
Extra virgin olive oil

Directions

1. Season salmon with salt and pepper, bake on 400 degrees for 10-15 minutes.

2. Chop onions and leeks.

3. Mince garlic and ginger.

4. Chop broccoli and mushrooms into bite size pieces.

5. Heat oil in pot.

6. Sauté onions, garlic, ginger and leek for about 2 minutes. Stir a few times while cooking.

7. Add 4 cups of filtered water and bring to boil.

8. Reduce heat to low.

9. Add broccoli, mushrooms, and seaweed.

10. Simmer about 3-5 minutes.

11. Turn off heat.

12. In each serving bowl add 1 tablespoon of miso.

13. Take a ladle and pour into each bowl one ladleful of hot soup.

14. Stir miso to blend evenly.

15. Fill the bowl full of soup broth, but not to the brim.

16. Place large pieces of salmon into each bowl on top.

Recipe Checklist for Miso Soup with Wild Alaskan Salmon

- Skill Level Required-Medium
- Ease of Preparation Grade-C+
- Speed of Preparation Grade-C
- Protein Grade-A
- Low Calorie-Yes
- Number of Nutritional Superstars-10
- Raw, Cooked or Both-Cooked
- Good for Entertaining-Yes

Recipe Wrap-Up

Serving wild Alaskan salmon to all your guests at a large party might be a little cost prohibitive, but this recipe will no doubt be a big hit. For dieters, the Miso Soup with Wild Alaskan Salmon recipe is a fantastic pick as it is high in protein and omega-3 fatty acids. Further, this recipe has a host of nutrition superstars like broccoli, miso, shitake mushrooms, seaweed, ginger and garlic.

Wild Alaskan Salmon Chowder with Yams

Serves 2-3

This salmon chowder is decidedly healthier and lighter than the traditional heavy cream chowders we are used to. It has a delicious sweet flavor and will likely become one of your winter favorites.

Ingredients

1 Tablespoon olive oil
¾ of a pound of Wild Alaskan Salmon
3 cloves of garlic
1 onion
Red bell pepper
2 small to medium size yams
Lime
Salt
Pepper
Cayenne Pepper
1 bay leaf
½ cup almond milk or soymilk

Directions

1. Chop onions and garlic.

2. Chop sweet potatoes into cubes.

3. Add olive oil to pot.

4. Sauté onions and garlic.

5. Add yam cubes, 1-teaspoon salt, soymilk or almond milk, and 1 bay leaf.

6. Bring to boil, and then simmer for 15 minutes.

7. Remove bay leaf.

8.   Dice red pepper.

9.   Add to the pot the salmon, red pepper, juice of 1 lime, 1 teaspoon of cayenne pepper. (Also add extra nut milk if needed.)

10. Cook on medium heat for 8 minutes.

11. Season with salt, pepper and cayenne pepper as needed.

Recipe Checklist for Wild Alaskan Salmon Chowder with Yams

- Skill Level Required-Medium
- Ease of Preparation Grade-C+
- Speed of Preparation Grade-C
- Protein Grade-A
- Low Calorie-A
- Number of Nutritional Superstars-10
- Raw, Cooked or Both-Cooked
- Good For Entertaining-Yes

Recipe Wrap-Up

Wild Alaskan Salmon Chowder with Yams will probably delight most dieters as the recipe is fairly novel. The much-overlooked yam gets some attention in this dish.

Wild Alaskan Salmon with Basil Portobello Mushrooms

Serves 2

This salmon dish is very easy and simple to prepare. You can use a variety of different types of mushrooms. Try combining some new ones you have never tried before in addition or instead of the basic button mushrooms. Good choices for this recipe are Portobello's, baby Portobello's, and shitakes. If you don't have fresh basil, you can also substitute fresh parsley for a new delicious twist.

Ingredients

2 Tablespoons extra virgin olive oil
¾ of a pound of Wild Alaskan Salmon
3 cloves of garlic
Lemon
1-½ cups of mushrooms

½ cup of basil
Salt
Pepper
Cayenne Pepper

Directions

1. Preheat oven to 400F.

2. Season salmon with salt and pepper.

3. Add a dash of olive oil to cover the pan.

4. Cook salmon on medium temperature for 8-10 minutes. Salmon will be opaque when ready.

5. Turn salmon over after 4 minutes.

6. Dice mushrooms into small pieces.

7. Chop basil roughly.

8. Chop garlic.

9. Add 1-tablespoon olive oil to pan.

10. Add garlic and mushrooms and sauté.

11. Add juice of half a lemon, 1-teaspoon salt and 1 teaspoon cayenne powder.

12. Cook for about 3 minutes.

13. Wilt basil over mushrooms.

14. Stir well

15. Place mushrooms on the bottom of each plate.

16. Serve fish on top of mushrooms.

17. Serve with a wedge of lemon.

18. Season fish with more salt and pepper as needed.

Recipe Checklist for Wild Alaskan Salmon with Basil Portobello Mushrooms

- Skill Level Required-Medium
- Ease of Preparation Grade-C
- Speed of Preparation Grade-C
- Protein Grade-A
- Low Calorie-Yes

- Number of Nutritional Superstars-(Only salt and pepper don't make the list.)
- Raw, Cooked or Both-Cooked
- Good For Entertaining-Maybe (It depends on your skill level in the kitchen.)

Recipe Wrap-Up

The Wild Alaskan Salmon with Portobello Mushrooms is a fine example of how a few simple ingredients treated well can be a real treat. If you have never had salmon and Portobello mushrooms before then you will certainly enjoy this great salmon dish.

You may not eat sardines very often but the bottom line is that you most definitely should. Many nutritionist and health experts feel that sardines are one of the more nutritious foods that you can eat. Why? The simple sardine is low on the food chain and that means that it is thus lower in mercury and other heavy metals when compared to other fish. But this is just the beginning of why sardines are so great. Sardines are also high in omega-3 fatty acids, low in calories and high in protein. In short, if you are on a diet, then sardines should be a food that you learn to like.

Spicy Sardine Pasta

Serves 2

This sardine dish is extremely simple to make quickly. If you are on a gluten free diet, you can make the same dish without the breadcrumbs. This recipe always turns out well either way.

Ingredients

1 Tablespoon extra virgin olive oil
3.75 oz tin of sardines
4 cloves of garlic
Brown rice pasta
Salt
½ cup breadcrumbs
Red Pepper Flakes
Parsley
Pepper

Directions

1. Boil water and prepare brown rice pasta.

2. Chop garlic cloves.

3. Heat olive oil in pan.

4. Sauté garlic.

5. Add breadcrumbs, stir, and cook 1-2 minutes. Make sure breadcrumbs get slightly toasted but not brown or burnt.

6. Drain sardines and add them to pan.

7. Add 1-teaspoon red pepper flakes, 1-teaspoon salt, 1-teaspoon pepper and 1-teaspoon parsley.

8. Cook 3-4 minutes while stirring.

9. Mix pasta in with sardine mixture.

10. Season as needed with additional salt and pepper.

Recipe Checklist for Spicy Sardine Pasta

- Skill Level Required-Medium
- Ease of Preparation Grade-B-
- Speed of Preparation Grade-B
- Protein Grade-A
- Low Calorie-A
- Number of Nutritional Superstars-5 (Olive oil, sardines, garlic, pepper flakes and parsley.)
- Raw, Cooked or Both-Cooked
- Good For Entertaining-Maybe (Better check ahead of time to see if your friends like or are willing to try sardines.)

Recipe Wrap-Up

Sardines are just great for you and an exceptional food for dieters. If you don't like sardines, try giving them a chance. Try different recipes and different brands of sardines before giving up.

Curry Tomato Sardines with Brown Rice

Serves 2

This is a spicy sardine recipe that has very bold flavors. It is a mix of a traditional Mediterranean style with a touch of Indian from the curry powder. You will be surprised how well these flavors work together.

Ingredients

1 Tablespoons Extra Virgin olive oil
1 Red bell pepper
1 red onion
1-cup brown rice
1 leek
2 cloves garlic
1-cup mushrooms
1 zucchini
2 tins of sardines 3.75 oz
1 15 oz can of crushed tomatoes
1-tablespoon curry powder
Salt
Pepper
Red Pepper Flakes

Directions

1. Prepare brown rice.
2. Chop garlic, onions, leek, zucchini, red pepper and mushrooms.
3. Add olive oil to skillet.
4. Sauté garlic, onions, leek, zucchini, red pepper and mushrooms for 3-5 minutes. Cook until onions are translucent.
5. Remove vegetables from skillet and set aside.
6. Add tomatoes into skillet.
7. Drain and add sardines and 2 teaspoons red pepper flakes.
8. Simmer for 3-5 minutes.
9. Add vegetables back into pan.
10. Season with 1-teaspoon curry powder, salt and pepper.
11. Serve sardines over brown rice.

Recipe Checklist for Curry Tomato Sardines with Brown Rice

- Skill Level Required-Moderate
- Ease of Preparation Grade-B
- Speed of Preparation Grade-B
- Protein Grade-A
- Low Calorie-A
- Number of Nutritional Superstars-11 (All ingredients except for salt and pepper.)
- Raw, Cooked or Both-Cooked
- Good For Entertaining-Maybe (Check with your guests.)

Recipe Wrap-Up

This is a sardine dish that will seem very filling to most, but is still quite low calorie at the same time.

Chapter 22

RECIPES WITH LENTILS

One of the great things about lentils is there are so many different kinds available. Lentils contain protein including essential amino acids. Many people who are vegetarians opt for a great deal of lentils in their diet instead of meat. Lentils also have a lot of iron. This is another reason why they are great for vegetarians.

One great tip is to shop around extensively. As it turns out not all lentils are created equally as some are just more nutritious than others. With a little research you can find lentils that are a cut above the rest. Eden brands, for example, sell lentils that are generally higher in nutritional value than most other lentil brands. So read your labels and you will be rewarded.

Here are just a few of the types of lentils available:

French Green Lentils
Black Beluga Lentils
Green Lentils
Tan or Yellow Lentils
Masoor Lentils
Red Lentils
White Lentils

Black Beluga Lentil Recipes

Black beluga lentils are great because they are delicate and shiny. They are smaller than regular lentils and often more expensive. They are called black beluga lentils because when you cook them they look like black beluga caviar.

At first you may find that black beluga lentils are a bit difficult to find so you may need to look in a health food store. However, it is definitely worth the hassle as black beluga lentils are quite delicious and have a flavor all of their own.

Black Beluga Lentil Soup

Serves 2

This is a basic recipe that you should be able to make with ingredients that you already have in your kitchen. Black beluga lentil soup is a great meal on a cold day or when you want something nutritious but just don't have time to make a complex meal.

Ingredients

1 Onion
2 Cloves of Garlic
1 Carrot
1 Bay leaf
1 cup of black beluga lentils (rinsed)
1 Tablespoon extra virgin olive oil
Salt
Pepper
Cayenne Red Pepper
Parsley (dried or fresh)

Directions

1. Dice onion and garlic, set aside.

2. Peel and dice carrot.

3. Heat olive oil in a pot over a medium temperature. Add onion and garlic and cook until onion is tender.

4. Stir in bay leaf.

5. Stir in carrot and cook 2 minutes.

6. Stir black beluga lentils into the pot.

7. Add 2 cups of filtered water and bring to a boil.

8. Simmer for 20-30 minutes until lentils are tender.

9. Season with salt and pepper to taste.

10. Also add cayenne pepper and parsley on top of your soup for added flavor.

Recipe Checklist for Black Beluga Lentil Soup

- Skill Level Required-Medium

- Ease of Preparation Grade-B

- Speed of Preparation Grade-B

- Protein Grade-B

- Low Calorie-A

- Number of Nutritional Superstars-8 (Onion, garlic, carrot, bay leaf, lentils, olive oil, cayenne pepper, parsley)

- Raw, Cooked or Both-Cooked with some raw elements

- Good For Entertaining-Yes (Due to the fact that this recipe is so basic, you should be able to serve it for a party.)

Recipe Wrap-Up

Part of this recipes charm is that it is a great low-calorie recipe that is extremely filling as well. You will likely make this recipe over and over.

Salad with Black Beluga Lentils

Serves 4

You might not typically think about lentils in salad, but they black beluga lentils actually complement the taste of a salad very well. One of the reasons black beluga lentils go so well in a salad is that they tend to hold their shape better after cooking than other lentils. They add a great deal of protein into your vegetables and compliment the taste at the same time. This salad with black beluga lentils is a perfect lunch.

Ingredients

1 cup black beluga lentils (rinsed)
1 red onion
2 red peppers
2 cups cherry tomatoes
1 cucumber
Extra virgin olive oil
Handful of fresh rosemary
Handful of fresh parsley
One lemon

2 cloves of garlic
Salt
Red Cayenne Pepper
Pepper

Directions

1. Bring black beluga lentils and 2 cups of water to boil.

2. Add a teaspoon of salt.

3. Simmer for 20-30 minutes until water is absorbed and lentils are tender.

4. Take lentils off stove and chill 2-3 hours.

5. Chop garlic and add to large mixing bowl.

6. Dice red peppers, cucumber and cherry tomatoes and add to bowl.

7. Chop rosemary and parsley and add to salad.

8. Pour black beluga lentils into the bowl.

9. Add about 1 tablespoon of olive oil.

10. Squeeze lemon into bowl.

11. Toss all ingredients.

12. Season with salt, pepper and cayenne pepper.

Recipe Checklist for Salad with Black Beluga Lentils

- Skill Level Required-Low
- Ease of Preparation Grade-A-
- Speed of Preparation Grade-B
- Protein Grade-B
- Low Calorie-A
- Number of Nutritional Superstars-11
- Raw, Cooked or Both-Both
- Good For Entertaining-Yes

Recipe Wrap-Up

How can you possibly go wrong with a recipe that is this full of great ingredients? The answer of course is that you can't! The Salad with Black Beluga Lentils recipe is definitely a sure fire winner, just give it a try.

Red Lentil Recipes

Red lentils have a taste that is very similar to black lentils but not identical. When you are in the mood for a change of pace, these recipes are a great idea. Red lentils are will work well in all sorts of dishes including those that have a sweet component such as Red Lentil Soup with Apricots.

Red Lentil Soup with Apricots

Serves 6

Ingredients

1 cup red lentils
½ cup dried apricots
1 onion
2 cups cherry tomatoes
Extra virgin olive oil
Handful of fresh parsley
½ lemon
2 cloves of garlic
5 cups of organic chicken broth or organic vegetable broth
Salt
Red Cayenne Pepper
Pepper
1 teaspoon Cumin

Directions

1. Heat oil in pot.

2. Sauté garlic and onions until onion is limp.

3. Add cumin to pot and stir.

4. Add lentils to the pot.

5. Add organic chicken soup or vegetable soup broth.

6. Bring to boil.

7. Simmer on slow for 20-30 minutes or until lentils are tender.

8. Stir in tomatoes and apricots.

9. Cook soup on low temperature for 5 more minutes

10. Take soup off heat and squeeze in ½ lemon.

11. Season with salt, pepper, cayenne pepper and parsley.

Recipe Checklist for Red Lentil Soup with Apricots

- Skill Level Required-Moderate
- Ease of Preparation Grade-B
- Speed of Preparation Grade-B-
- Protein Grade-B
- Low Calorie-Yes
- Number of Nutritional Superstars-10 (Lentils, apricots, onion, tomatoes, olive oil, parsley, lemon, garlic, cayenne pepper and cumin.)
- Raw, Cooked or Both-Cooked
- Good For Entertaining-Maybe (The time involved in cooking this dish isn't excessive but it may not be perfect for all entertaining situations.)

Recipe Wrap-Up

When you want a change of pace, this is a simply perfect recipe. Most have never had a dish quite like the Red Lentil Soup with Apricot. For this reason it is very memorable, especially the first few times.

Pasta with Lentil Sauce

Serves 6

Ingredients

Brown rice pasta
1-cup brown lentils
1 onion
3 cloves garlic
Extra virgin olive oil
Red pepper flakes
Salt
Pepper
1-cup tomatoes
Parsley (fresh or dried)

Directions

1. Heat 1 tsp. oil in pot.
2. Sauté garlic and onions until onion is limp.

3. Add lentils and 2 ½ cups of filtered water.

4. Bring water to boil and simmer lentils for about 20 minutes.

5. Prepare brown rice pasta according to directions.

6. Drain pasta and set aside.

7. One lentils are firm, add in tomatoes and one teaspoon of red pepper flakes and stir.

8. Add pasta into the lentil mixture.

9. Season with salt and pepper

10. Add fresh or dried parsley to the top of this dish.

Recipe Checklist for Pasta with Lentil Sauce

- Skill Level Required-Medium
- Ease of Preparation Grade-B+
- Speed of Preparation Grade-B
- Protein Grade-B
- Low Calorie-Yes
- Number of Nutritional Superstars-7 (Lentils, onion, garlic, live oil, red pepper flakes, tomatoes, parsley)
- Raw, Cooked or Both-Cooked
- Good For Entertaining-Yes (This recipe is designed to feed six people and will also work very well for vegans and vegetarians.

Recipe Wrap-Up

Pasta with Lentil Sauce should bring a smile to your face. This recipe is simple, but heavy on flavor with lots of garlic, parsley and red pepper flakes.

The fact that this recipe is high in protein and low in calories should make it one that dieters will turn to again and again.

Curry of Red Lentils

Serves 4

Ingredients

- 1 cup red lentils
- 1 red onion
- 1 Tablespoon coconut oil
- 2 Tablespoons curry powder
- 1 Tablespoon fresh ginger
- 3 cloves of garlic
- 1-teaspoon turmeric
- 1-teaspoon cayenne pepper
- 1 small can of tomato paste
- 1-cup brown basmati rice
- ¼ cup cilantro

Directions

1. Rinse lentils and put them in a pot with 2 cups of water.
2. Bring lentils and water to boil.
3. Reduce cooking temperature to simmer.
4. Cook for about 20 minutes until lentils are tender.
5. Prepare brown basmati rice.
6. Chop garlic and mince the ginger root.
7. Sauté onions in a pan with coconut oil.
8. Once onions have wilted, add all spices including garlic and ginger.
9. Cook for 1-2 minutes on medium-low temperature stirring spices into onions.
10. Add tomato paste to pan and continue to cook on medium-low.
11. When lentils are tender, drain them and add to pan.
12. Stir lentils into the curry mixture.
13. Roughly chop cilantro.
14. Serve brown rice with the curry of red lentils.
15. Top generously with cilantro.

Recipe Checklist for Curry of Red Lentils

- Skill Level Required-Medium
- Ease of Preparation Grade-C
- Speed of Preparation Grade-C
- Protein Grade-B
- Low Calorie-B (This dish is low calorie so long as you don't go overboard on the coconut oil.)
- Number of Nutritional Superstars-11
- Raw, Cooked or Both-Cooked, but with some raw elements.
- Good For Entertaining-Maybe (Whether or not you want to tackle this recipe depends upon your skill in the kitchen. One fact is for certain, however; your guests will love this meal.)

Recipe Wrap-Up

Curry of Red Lentils is a dish with a lot of taste. The mixture of spices should be enough to get anyone's attention. If you really want to make this dish memorable consider loading on the cilantro.

Chapter 23
NUT AND SEEDS RECIPES

Medical studies and science have shown us repeatedly that one of the very best foods you can eat are nuts and seeds. There are a variety of reasons that nuts and seeds are so fantastic for you and they, of course, differ nutritionally by the type of nut and seed. In general, however, nuts and seeds are high in protein, minerals, vitamins and even fiber. Nuts and seeds are easy to transport, won't spoil and provide serious nutrition. Squirrels love nuts for a good reason!

Walnuts

We will be spending a lot of time on walnuts and almonds in this chapter. Both of these nuts are nutritional superstars that you will love even more than you already do once you know all the facts. Walnuts, for example, are rich in omega-3 fatty acids, which are extremely good for brain and heart health.

Almonds

Almonds, much like walnuts, are also high in nutrition and protein. Almonds, once again like walnuts, have been shown to be beneficial to brain health.

The good news about nuts in general is that they are a fine source of protein and vitamins and some nuts such as chestnuts are even low in fat. Dieters do have to be aware of the fat and calorie content of nuts and seeds in general, with the one notable expectation being chestnuts, which are generally lower in both fat and calories. However, nuts and seeds in general are a wonderful way to get easily digested protein and lots of vitamins and minerals as a bonus.

Here are some great walnut, almond and seed recipes that should please dieters quite a bit. Remember that walnuts and almonds are two of the healthier nuts that you can eat and you can enjoy them in moderation year round.

Walnut Recipes

Brown Rice Pasta with Walnut Pesto

Serves 4

Ingredients

    Brown rice pasta
    Extra virgin olive oil
    ½ cup fresh parsley
    6 garlic cloves
    1 Lemon
    1-cup fresh basil
    ½ cup walnuts
    Salt
    Pepper
    Cayenne Pepper

Directions

1. Prepare brown rice pasta according to directions. Set aside.
2. Blend the 6 garlic cloves in the food processor.
3. Add in the following ingredients: Parsley, Basil, walnuts, squeeze of lemon, 1 tablespoon extra virgin olive oil and a teaspoon of salt.
4. Blend until pesto is smooth.
5. Toss pesto sauce with pasta.
6. Season with pepper and cayenne pepper.

Recipe Checklist for Brown Rice Pasta with Walnut Pesto

- Skill Level Required-Moderate
- Ease of Preparation Grade-B
- Speed of Preparation Grade-B
- Protein Grade-A
- Low Calorie-B
- Number of Nutritional Superstars-7 (Olive oil, parsley, garlic, lemon, basil, walnuts and cayenne pepper)
- Raw, Cooked or Both-Raw
- Good For Entertaining-Yes

Recipe Wrap-Up

Its hard to go wrong with the Brown Rice Pasta with Walnut Pesto as you are getting protein from both the brown rice pasta and the walnuts at the same time. This is one of those dishes that is sure to go over well with vegans and vegetarians as it is high in protein and flavor.

Cranberry, Cherry and Walnut Salad

Serves 4

Ingredients

Extra virgin olive oil
Lemon
¼ cup dried cranberries
¼ cup dried cherries
3 cups baby spinach
¼ cup goat cheese
¼ cup fresh basil
1 clove garlic
½ cup walnuts
Salt
Pepper
Cayenne Pepper

Directions

1. Combine 2 tablespoons extra virgin olive oil, juice of one lemon, 2-tablespoons of cranberries, 1 clove garlic and 1-teaspoon salt into the food processor.

2. Process until smooth.

3. Add remaining ingredients into a salad bowl.

4. Pour dressing on top and toss.

5. Season with salt and pepper as needed.

Recipe Checklist for Cranberry, Cherry and Walnut Salad

- Skill Level Required-Moderate
- Ease of Preparation Grade-B

- Speed of Preparation Grade-B
- Protein Grade-A
- Low Calorie-B
- Number of Nutritional Superstars-9 (This recipe scores a 9 as it has cranberries, cherries, spinach, basil, garlic, walnuts and cayenne pepper)
- Raw, Cooked or Both-Raw
- Good For Entertaining-Yes

Recipe Wrap-Up

Your friends will love the Cranberry, Cherry and Walnut Salad as it has a great amount of flavor and nutrition. Due to the fact that this tasty salad also has goat cheese, you can expect a higher overall level of protein. The cranberries and cherries work to provide the dish with a boost of vitamin C, and these two fruits will contrast nicely with the fresh basil and spinach. In short, this dish is a winner!

Almond Recipes

Here are some great almond recipes that you are sure to love. Once you've tried them all you will no doubt be hooked on the taste of almonds.

Broccoli Stir Fry with Almonds

Serves 8

*Note this recipe is designed to be vegetarian, but you can add organic meat to the recipe with great results.

Ingredients

2 cups Brown rice
Extra virgin olive oil
10 cups of fresh broccoli
3 garlic cloves
1 Lemon
Fresh ginger
½ cup chopped almonds
Lemon
Tamari soy sauce
Salt

Pepper

Cayenne Pepper

Directions

1. Put 1 Tablespoon extra virgin olive oil into a pan or wok.

2. Stir-fry broccoli for about 2 minutes until still very green and crisp.

3. Mince ginger and chop garlic cloves.

4. Stir into the pan the garlic, ginger and ¼ cup soy sauce.

5. Cook for 1 minute.

6. Remove from heat.

7. Stir in almonds and 1 big squeeze of fresh lemon.

8. Serve with brown rice.

9. Modification with meat (prepare the meat once you have completed the other directions.)

10. Cut meat into thin strips.

11. Add another Tablespoon of extra virgin olive oil to pan.

12. Add 2 more chopped cloves of garlic.

13. Sautee cloves for about 30 seconds.

14. Add meat to pan and sauté until it is cooked through.

15. Season with salt, pepper and cayenne pepper.

16. Serve with Broccoli Stir Fry with Almonds.

Recipe Checklist for Broccoli Stir Fry with Almonds

- Skill Level Required-Medium

- Ease of Preparation Grade-B

- Speed of Preparation Grade-B

- Protein Grade-C

- Low Calorie-Yes (Just don't put in too many almonds or too much oil.)

- Number of Nutritional Superstars-8 (Olive oil, broccoli, garlic, lemon, ginger, almonds, ginger and cayenne pepper)

- Raw, Cooked or Both-Cooked

- Good For Entertaining-Yes (This is definitely a great one for a small party or get together as the recipe is designed to serve up to eight people.)

Recipe Wrap-Up

Broccoli is back, and this time it is paired with almonds. This delightful recipe is designed to make the most out of the way stir-fry blends together the various flavors. In particular, you will notice that in this recipe the cayenne pepper, garlic, almonds and broccoli interplay nicely.

Almond Quinoa

Serves 4

Ingredients

1-cup quinoa
Extra virgin olive oil
½ cup dried cherries
½ cup chopped almonds or slivered almonds
1 yellow or red bell pepper
2 garlic cloves
2 scallions
1 Zucchini
Thyme (fresh or dried)
Salt
Pepper
Cayenne Pepper
Lemon

Directions

1.   Rinse Quinoa

2.   Chop yellow pepper into small chunks.

3.   Mince garlic and dice scallions.

4.   Dice zucchini into small pieces.

5.   In saucepan, heat 1 tablespoon of extra virgin olive oil.

6.   Add pepper, garlic and scallions and cook for about 5 minutes.

7.   Stir in quinoa, 2 cups of water, 2 teaspoons of thyme and 1-teaspoon salt.

8.   Bring mixture to boil.

9.   Reduce to simmer and cook for 8 minutes.

10.   Stir zucchini into the pot.

11.   Cook for 5 minutes more.

12. Stir in almonds and 2 more teaspoons of extra virgin olive oil.

13. Let cool

14. Squeeze lemon or lime over quinoa before serving.

Recipe Checklist for Almond Quinoa

- Skill Level Required-Moderate

- Ease of Preparation Grade-B-

- Speed of Preparation Grade-C

- Protein Grade-A (The combination of quinoa and almonds means that this dish has a lot of protein.)

- Low Calorie-Yes (Just don't overdo the nuts.)

- Number of Nutritional Superstars-12 (Every ingredient except salt and pepper fall into the nutritional superstar category. In a word there are no empty calories in this recipe, so enjoy!)

- Raw, Cooked or Both-Cooked

- Good For Entertaining-Maybe (If you are an experienced cook then this might work for you, but less experienced cooks might want to look at another recipe for entertaining or trying to impress that special someone.)

Recipe Wrap-Up

Quinoa is an ingredient that not too many people are familiar with, but it is very nutritious and has been used for thousands a years. It is recommended that you rinse your quinoa before you begin cooking with it.

Almond Milk

Almond milk is a great alternative to regular milk. You can buy it in the grocery store, but the almond milk that is typically sold has added sweeteners. It can also really add up in costs. A great alternative is to make your own almond milk.

Almond Milk

Ingredients

1 cup of almonds
4 cups of filtered water
Nut milk bag

Directions

1. Combine almonds and water in a large covered container.

2. Soak the almonds overnight.

3. Come morning, blend almonds and water in a blender. Keep blending until you hear the rattling stop.

4. Strain the milk through a nut milk bag; this will filter out the fibers from the milk.

5. The great news is that you can actually use this same recipe with different nuts including walnuts, cashew and macadamia nut. You could also use sunflower or sesame seed milk.

6. Another variation on this recipe is that you can add dates, agave or vanilla for added sweetener.

Recipe Wrap-Up

Making your own almond milk is pretty simple once you've gotten the hand of it. The fact is there is little reason to buy cartons of almond milk when you can have your own fresh almond milk waiting in the refrigerator for less money.

Pumpkin Seed Recipes

Pumpkin seeds are nutritional wonders full of vitamins, minerals and protein. Try and work pumpkin seeds into your diet at least one a week and remember they make great snacks too.

Pumpkin Soup Topped with Pumpkin Seeds

Serves 8

Ingredients

Extra virgin olive oil
One leek
2 cloves of garlic
1 apple
½ tsp. Cinnamon
½ tsp. Ginger
2 cans of pumpkin
1 can organic chicken broth (vegetable broth can be substituted)

1-cup soymilk
Pumpkin seeds
Salt
Pepper
Cayenne pepper

Directions

1. Chop the garlic and leek.

2. Heat 1 Tablespoon of olive oil and sauté the garlic and leek.

3. Add cinnamon and ginger and stir into mixture. Let cook for about 1 minute.

4. Dice the apple.

5. Add chopped apple to pot and cook for another 2 minutes.

6. Add 1 can chicken broth and also add 2 cups of filtered water.

7. Bring to boil and then turn down heat to simmer for 15 minutes.

8. Stir in pumpkin and soymilk while stirring constantly.

9. Cook on low temperature for five minutes.

10. Season with salt, pepper and cayenne pepper.

11. Top with pumpkin seeds.

Recipe Checklist for Pumpkin Soup Topped with Pumpkin Seeds

- Skill Level Required-Moderate
- Ease of Preparation Grade-B
- Speed of Preparation Grade-B
- Protein Grade-A
- Low Calorie-B
- Number of Nutritional Superstars-9 (Olive oil, leeks, garlic, apple, cinnamon, ginger, pumpkin, pumpkin seeds and cayenne pepper.)
- Raw, Cooked or Both-Cooked and Raw
- Good For Entertaining-Yes

Recipe Wrap-Up

Pumpkin is low in calories but pumpkin seeds are not. The combination of both pumpkins and pumpkin seeds provide for a nice nutritional spread that helps make this a great meal for dieters.

Chapter 24

RECIPES FEATURING BROCCOLI

Broccoli is, simply stated, a food that you most definitely want to eat and eat often. The facts are that broccoli is nutritious and so good for you that eating it everyday may not be that bad of an idea. In the world of veggies, broccoli standouts amongst even its more nutritional peers.

You may have heard people state that they don't want to eat broccoli. Why you might even fall into this category, but broccoli has so much to offer you in terms of health and dieting that you really should consider this impressive veggie. Broccoli can effectively fill up almost any stomach. If you are skeptical of this fact, just eat three hundred calories of broccoli and see if you are full!

Just a few hundred grams of broccoli, or roughly 3.5 ounces, is loaded down with all sorts of vitamins and minerals. While many people realize that broccoli is good for them, they probably don't realize just how good for them it is. Broccoli has about 150% of one's daily requirement of vitamin C, which is far higher than one could expect. Broccoli also has several B vitamins, calcium, vitamin A, zinc, magnesium, potassium, iron and calcium, but this is only the beginning of what broccoli can offer.

Broccoli Has A Special Surprise For You

Study after study shows that broccoli contains compounds that fight all kinds of diseases and cancers. Compounds in broccoli have been shown to boost the immune system and broccoli works as an anti-viral and anti-bacterial as well. Moreover, these chemicals seem to withstand most forms of storage and preparation very well, meaning that you can steam, freeze and prepare broccoli in almost any fashion and it will retain its nutritional and disease fighting properties. If you want truly want to be healthy, you should find a way of getting broccoli onto your plate and the plates of your family.

Simple Broccoli Soup

Serves 2

Ingredients

    Extra virgin olive oil
One onion
1 Bay leaf
1 Red bell pepper
5 cups of broccoli
3 cups of vegetable broth
Salt
Pepper
Cayenne Pepper

Directions:

1. Dice onion.
2. Put 1 Tablespoon of extra virgin olive oil in pot.
3. Add chopped onion and 1 bay leaf and sauté until onion is translucent.
4. Chop broccoli and bell pepper.
5. Add the broccoli and pepper to the pot along with vegetable broth and 1-cup water.
6. Bring to boil, and then reduce to a simmer for 8 minutes, stirring occasionally.
7. Remove Bay leaf.
8. Season with salt and pepper.
9. Top with florets of broccoli.
10. Season with salt, pepper, and red pepper.

Recipe Checklist for Simple Broccoli Soup

Skill Level Required-Low

- Ease of Preparation Grade-B
- Speed of Preparation Grade-C+
- Protein Grade-C
- Low Calorie-Yes
- Number of Nutritional Superstars-Five (Olive oil, pepper, broccoli, cayenne pepper, onions)

- Raw, Cooked or Both-Cooked
- Good For Entertaining-Yes (Good for vegetarian and vegan guests)

Recipe Wrap-Up

The fact that this recipe is simple and relatively easy to prepare helps make it a winner. Considering that it also has olive oil and bell peppers in addition to broccoli definitely makes it a nutritious meal. The wide array of health benefits offered by this combination is a good reason to add it to your diet.

Dieters should be happy with the simple broccoli soup, as it is quite low in calories, especially if you go light on the olive oil. Remember olive oil, while very nutritious, is also high in calories.

Raw Broccoli Salad

Serves 2

Ingredients

3 cups of chopped broccoli
2 cloves of garlic
1 tsp of cumin seeds
Extra virgin olive oil
1 Red or yellow pepper
1/8-cup fresh basil
Two roma tomatoes
Hemp seeds
1 cup of chopped spinach
Salt
Pepper

Directions

1. Finely chop the broccoli.

2. Mince the garlic.

3. Add together the following in a large bowl: broccoli, garlic, 1/8 cup olive oil, cumin seeds, juice from one lemon and 1 teaspoon salt.

4. Mix thoroughly.

5. Put in refrigerator for 45 minutes.

6. Chop bell pepper and tomato.

7. Once you have removed the broccoli mixture from the refrigerator, add in chopped pepper and tomato. Mix well.

8. Add 1-teaspoon hemp seeds, and pepper to taste.

Recipe Checklist for Raw Broccoli Salad

- Skill Level Required-Low

- Ease of Preparation Grade-A

- Speed of Preparation Grade-B

- Protein Grade-B (Hemp seeds are high in protein)

- Low Calorie-Yes (Just go light on the olive oil.)

- Number of Nutritional Superstars-9

- Raw, Cooked or Both-Raw

- Good For Entertaining Yes (Good for vegetarian and vegan guests)

Recipe Wrap-Up

Raw Broccoli Salad consists of not less than nine different nutritional superstars, which means that adding it to your recipe list is really a no-brainer. Likewise since the Raw Broccoli Salad is raw, as the name indicates, you will be getting all the valuable enzymes and nutrients that cooking can remove from food. It's a dish that will also make your vegetarian and vegan friends quite happy, as it is both tasty and quite nutritious.

If you are in a rush, especially for impromptu entertaining, this is a great dish to consider. While one is technically supposed to let the Raw Broccoli Salad chill for about 45 minutes, this isn't absolutely necessary. Of course, this means that the Raw Broccoli Salad can be prepared quickly when needed.

Sweet Broccoli Salad

Serves 2

Ingredients

3 cups of chopped broccoli
¾ cup raisins
¾ cup dried cranberries

1 red onion
1 red or yellow pepper
¾ cup celery
¼ cup sunflower seeds
¼ cup pumpkin seeds
Extra virgin olive oil
Fresh lemon
Salt
Pepper

Directions:

1. Chop the broccoli into small pieces.

2. Chop red onion, pepper and celery,

3. Add the following into a mixing bowl: broccoli, raisins, cranberries, and celery.

4. Top with 1 tablespoon olive oil.

5. Squeeze one lemon into bowl.

6. Add one-teaspoon salt and one-teaspoon pepper.

7. Toss salad to mix thoroughly.

8. Add in raisins, cranberries, sunflower and pumpkin seeds.

9. Mix again and serve.

Recipe Checklist for Sweet Broccoli Salad

*   Skill Level Required-Low

*   Ease of Preparation Grade A

*   Speed of Preparation Grade B

*   Protein Grade B (Sunflower and pumpkin seeds have a good amount of protein)

*   Low Calorie-That depends mainly on the amount of seeds you put into the salad

*   Number of Nutritional Superstars-10 (All the ingredients other than salt and pepper.)

*   Raw, Cooked or Both-Raw

*   Good For Entertaining-Yes (Good for vegetarians and vegans guests.)

Recipe Wrap-Up

If you are looking for a broccoli salad that has a little bit more protein, then you can't go wrong with the Sweet Broccoli Salad. The Sweet Broccoli Salad, due to the fact that it has sunflower and pumpkin seeds, also means that it has a good deal of protein as well. Just be sure that you don't go to heavy on the seeds. While very nutrition and healthy, seeds are also high in calories.

The fact that this broccoli salad is also raw will please vegetarians and vegans alike. Consider substituting the Sweet Broccoli Salad for an animal protein dish once a week.

Roasted Broccoli

Serves 4

Ingredients

> 3 cups of chopped broccoli
> Extra virgin olive oil
> ½ cup pine nuts
> Fresh lemon
> Salt
> Pepper

Directions:

1. Heat over to 400F.

2. Separate broccoli into florets

3. Toss broccoli with 1-tablespoon olive oil, salt and pepper.

4. Spread broccoli out in a glass pan.

5. Bake for 10 minutes.

6. Sprinkle fresh lemon juice and pine nuts on broccoli.

Recipe Checklist for Roasted Broccoli

- Skill Level Required-Low

- Ease of Preparation Grade-A (Recipes don't get too much easier than this one.)

- Speed of Preparation Grade-B

- Protein Grade-C
- Low Calorie-Yes, you can always reduce the amount of olive oil.
- Number of Nutritional Superstars-3 (Broccoli, olive oil and lemon)
- Raw, Cooked or Both-Cooked
- Good For Entertaining-Yes (Roasted Broccoli Salad is great for entertaining. This dish looks like far more work than it is and your guest should love it.)

Indian Broccoli with Cauliflower

Serves 4

Ingredients

2 cups of broccoli
1 cup of cauliflower
1 red onion
1-cup cherry tomatoes
1-teaspoon chili powder
½ teaspoon garam masala
½ teaspoon cumin seeds
2 cloves of garlic
Fresh ginger
Coconut oil
Salt
Pepper

Directions:

1. Separate the broccoli and cauliflower into florets.
2. Dice garlic and grate 1 tablespoon of ginger.
3. Boil a pot of water and add broccoli and cauliflower.
4. Reduce to simmer after 3-5 minutes.
5. Drain water and set broccoli and cauliflower aside.
6. Add 1 tablespoon of coconut oil to pan.
7. Add cumin seeds and cook for 30 seconds.
8. Add onions and cook over medium heat until onions are brown.

9. Add tomato and cook for 2 minutes.

10. Put the chili powder, garam masala, garlic and ginger into the pan.

11. Cook for 2 minutes stirring well.

12. Combine broccoli and cauliflower with the spices. Be sure to mix thoroughly.

Recipe Checklist for Indian Broccoli with Cauliflower

- Skill Level Required-Medium
- Ease of Preparation Grade-B
- Speed of Preparation Grade-B
- Protein Grade-C
- Low Calorie-Yes
- Number of Nutritional Superstars-10
- Raw, Cooked or Both-Cooked
- Good For Entertaining-Yes (This meal is designed to serve several people.)

Recipe Wrap-Up

Part of what the Indian Broccoli with Cauliflower meal has going for it is that it sounds much more difficult to prepare than it is. But the fact is that this isn't too tough of a dish when contrasted against the final result. If you are looking for a dish that is relatively easy and will still impress, then this is a good one! Also, Indian Broccoli with Cauliflower has two vegetable stars in the recipe, which makes it a sure winner. Most people just don't eat enough broccoli or cauliflower, so this recipe is an easy and tasty way to get these two key vegetables and lots of healthy spices at the same time.

Broccoli and Tofu

Serves 2

Ingredients

2 cups of broccoli
1 onion
2 tablespoons extra virgin olive oil
1 block of firm tofu
2 tablespoons Tamari soy sauce
3 cloves of garlic

1-tablespoon fresh ginger
2 tablespoons sesame oil
2 tablespoons rice vinegar
2 teaspoons cornstarch
Salt
Pepper
Cayenne pepper

Directions:

1. In a small bowl, combine cayenne pepper, cornstarch, tamari, and sesame oil and rice vinegar.

2. Wisk together until blended well.

3. Chop onions and mince garlic.

4. Mince fresh ginger and set aside.

5. Put oil in a large skillet. Sauté onions and garlic until translucent.

6. Cut tofu into cubes,

7. Add tofu, ginger, and broccoli to the pan. Cook about 6 minutes.

8. Add the sauce to the broccoli and tofu.

9. Cook until sauce thickens.

Recipe Checklist for Broccoli and Tofu

- Skill Level Required-Medium
- Ease of Preparation Grade-B
- Speed of Preparation Grade-B
- Protein Grade-B
- Low Calorie-Yes
- Number of Nutritional Superstars-7 (Broccoli, onion, olive oil, tofu, garlic, ginger, cayenne pepper)
- Raw, Cooked or Both-Cooked
- Good For Entertaining-Yes

Recipe Wrap-Up

When you are looking for a recipe that is healthy but has lots of protein, then you can't go wrong with Broccoli and Tofu. If you are in the mood or need extra protein, then this recipe has a lot to offer. Of all the broccoli dishes offered in this chapter, the Broccoli and Tofu recipe works best as a low-calorie, high-protein meal. The protein level in this recipe can easily be increased to a high protein level by simply adding a bit more tofu.

Additionally, there are plenty of spices and garlic as well. Remember that garlic is one of the very best foods that you can eat. This recipe works quite well with extra garlic.

<Insert Steve Jones signature>

<Insert Frank Mangano signature>

ABOUT THE AUTHORS

Steve G. Jones

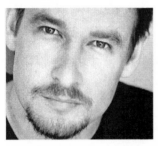 Steve G. Jones, M.Ed. is a board certified Clinical Hypnotherapist. He has been practicing hypnotherapy since the 1980s. He is the author of 22 books on Hypnotherapy. He is a member of the National Guild of Hypnotists, American Board of Hypnotherapy, president of the American Alliance of Hypnotists, on the board of directors of the Los Angeles chapter of the American Lung Association, and director of the California state registered Steve G. Jones School of Hypnotherapy. In order to keep up with the very latest in research, he regularly attends training conferences.

In the mid 80s, Steve began study at the University of Florida. His primary research focus was cognitive psychology, understanding how people learn. Much of is early research was published in psychology journals in the late 80s. Meanwhile, he continued practicing hypnosis outside of academia on a regular basis.

From 1990 to 1995, he was fortunate to counsel families and individuals. During this tie he finished his degree in psychology at the University of Florida and went on to graduate studies in counseling. He has a Bachelor's Degree in psychology from the University of Florida (1994), a Mater's Degree in education from Armstrong Atlantic State University (2007), and is currently working on a doctorate in education, Ed.D., at Georgia Southern University.

Steve G. Jones sees clients for a variety of conditions. Among them are: weight loss, anxiety, smoking cessation, test taking, phobias (such as fear of flying), nail biting, road rage, anger management, IBS, general wellness, pre-surgical and pre-dental pain control, natural childbirth, and many others. In business settings, he is regularly called upon by sales teams to boost salesperson motivation. His straightforward techniques have significantly and consistently increased sales. Steve G. Jones also works extensively with Hollywood actors, writers, directors, and producers, helping them achieve their very best.

http://www.BetterLivingWithHypnosis.com

Frank Mangano

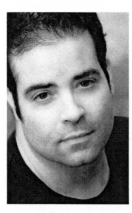

Frank Peter Mangano Jr. was born August 9th, 1977 in New York City where he still currently resides. Mangano is an American author, health advocate and independent researcher in the field of alternative health. He is the author of several books including *The 60 Day Prescription Free Cholesterol Cure*, *The Mind Killer Defense*, which he co-authored with Kim Wierman, *The Blood Pressure Miracle*, which continues to be a bestselling book on Amazon.com and *You Can Attract It*, which he co-authored with Steve G. Jones. Additionally, he has published numerous reports and a considerable amount of articles pertaining to natural health.

Mangano is an independent researcher and has no financial relationship to any pharmaceutical or supplements company. Therefore, his opinions are unbiased. He writes and researches health on a daily basis.

When asked when his interest in alternative medicine first began, he once responded by saying "Since as far back as I can remember prescription drugs always scared me. I always felt that if nature created a problem, it also had a solution." He started vitamin/mineral supplementation in his early teen years and now has a vast knowledge of how supplementation can be used to treat and prevent illnesses, diseases, ailments, infections, viruses and other health conditions. His insight is present in hundreds of articles related to this topic.

Mangano's strong passion for helping others improve their health inexpensively and naturally transformed into his full-time career and life mission when his mother was diagnosed with high cholesterol on the early 2000s. Her fear of the side effects associated with taking prescription drugs like statins led her to turn to him for help.

Determined to find a method for her to lower her cholesterol naturally, Mangano studied and reviewed medical books, reports, articles and case studies as well as literature on natural herbs, vitamins and minerals. After months of research, he synergistically combined all of his acquired knowledge and created a plan based on science that allowed her to lower her cholesterol without drugs. Her cholesterol dropped nearly 40 points with his all-natural system. Wanting to help more people, he wrote and self-published his first book called *The 60 Day Prescription-Free Cholesterol Cure*. The book is now helping numerous people worldwide lower their cholesterol naturally.

Mangano focuses a big portion of his time building and managing Natural Health On the Web, which offers readers free and valuable information on alternative remedies. The site currently contains information on an extensive amount of conditions, which can be treated & prevented using natural methods.

http://www.NaturalHealthOnTheWeb.com

REFERENCES

Bakalar, Nicholas. (2008). Symptoms: Metabolic Syndrome Is Tied to Diet Soda. *The New York Times.* Retrieved March 9, 2010 from http://www.nytimes.com/2008/02/05/health/nutrition/05symp.html.

Bass TM, Weinkove D, Houthofd K, Gems D, Partidge L. (2007). Effects of resveratrol on lifespan in Drosophila melanogaster and Caenorhabditis elegans. *Mechanisms of ageing and development.* 128 (10): 546-52.

Bernheim, Hippolyte. (1889). *Suggesting therapeutics: a treatise on the nature and use of hypnotism.* New York: Putnam Sons.

Breakstone, Stephanie. (2008). Newest soda danger discover the dangers of diet soda. *Prevention.* Retrieved from http://www.prevention.com/health/nutrition/healthy-eating-tips/soda-dangers/article.

Chang, Louse, MD. (2005). Meaty Diet May Raise Pancreatic Cancer Risk. *WebMD Health News.* Retrieved from http://www.webmd.com/food-recipes/news/20051004/meaty-diet-may-raise-pancreatic-cancer-risk.

Fain, Jean. (2004). You are getting thinner. *O, The Oprah Magazine.* 176-279.

Fletcher, Anne, MSRD. (2003). *Thin for life: 10 keys to success from people who have lsot weight and kept it off.* Boston: Houghton Miflin.

Gottlieb, Bill & Preuss, Harry, M.D. (2007). *The natural fat-loss pharmacy: drug-free remedies to help you safely lose weight.* New York: Broadway Books.

Goulding, Matt. (2009). The Best Worst and Best! Microwave Meals. *Men's Health.* Retrieved from http://eatthis.mensheath.com/content/worst-and-best-microwave-meals.

Goulding, Matt. (2009). The Twenty Worst Foods in America. *Men's Health.* Retrieved from http://www.menshealth.com/20worst/worstfood.html

Gurgevich, Steven. PH.d. (2008). Labor Pain Made Easy with Self-Hypnosis. *Psychology Today.* Retrieved from http://www.psychologytoday.com/blog/adventures-in-mind-body-medicine/200809/labor-pain-made-easier-self-hypnosis.Jeffers, S. (1989). *Feel the fear and do it anyway.* Rider & Co.

Jiang, R., Paik, D.C., Hankinson, JL, Barr, R.G. (2007). Cured meat consumption, lung function, and chronic obstructive pulmonary disease among United States adult. *American Journal of Respiratory and Critical Care Medicine.* Volume 175, Pages 798-80.

Jones, Steve, D. & Mangano, Frank. (2009). *You can attract it.* Connecticut: Strategic Book Publishing.

Kroger, William, S. (2007). *Clinical and experimental hypnosis: in medicine, dentistry and psychology.* Philadelphia: Lippincott Williams & Wilkins.

Ley-Jacobs, Beth & Sosin, Allen. (1998). *Alpha lipoic acid: nature's ultimate antioxidant.* New York: Kensington.

Mayo Clinic. (2007, January 9). Tips to Lose Weight and Keep It Off. *The Mayo Clinic Health Letter.* Retrieved March 9, 2010 from http://www.mayoclinic.org/news2007-mchi/3864.html.

Mercola, Joseph. (2005). Diet Sodas May Double Your Risk of Obesity. *Mercola.com.* Retrieved from http://articles.mercola.com/sites/articles/archive/2005/06/30/diet-sodas.aspx.

Reader's Digest. (2000). *The healing power of vitamins, minerals, and herbs.* Pleasantville: Readers Digest Books.

Schlosser, Eric. (2002). *Fast food nation: the dark side of the American meal.* New York: Houghton Mifflin.

Still, David. (2007). Can Red Wine Help You Live Forever? *Fortune Magazine.* Retrieved from http://money.cnn.com/2007/01/18/magazines/fortune/Live_forever.fortune/index.htm.

Trust for America's Health. (2009). F as in Fat, How Obesity Policies are Failing in America 2009. *Healthy Americans.* Retrieved from http://healthyamericans.org/reports/obesity2009.

Ulene, Valerie. (2008). Out of Control. *Los Angeles Times.* Retrieved from http://articles.latimes.com/2008/jan/21/health/he-themd21.

University of Exeter. (2009, October 26). Exercise Makes Cigarettes Less Attractive to Smokers. *ScienceDaily.* Retrieved March 9, 2010 from http://www. sciencedaily.com/releases/2009/10/091026093723.htm.

Wyshak, Grace. (2000). Consumption of Carbonated Drinks by Teenage Girls Associated with Bone Fractures. *Archives of Pediatrics & Adolescent Medicine.* 154:542-543,610-613.

BUY A SHARE OF THE FUTURE IN YOUR COMMUNITY

These certificates make great holiday, graduation and birthday gifts that can be personalized with the recipient's name. The cost of one S.H.A.R.E. or one square foot is $54.17. The personalized certificate is suitable for framing and will state the number of shares purchased and the amount of each share, as well as the recipient's name. The home that you participate in "building" will last for many years and will continue to grow in value.

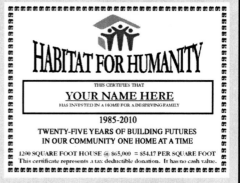

Here is a sample SHARE certificate:

YES, I WOULD LIKE TO HELP!

*I support the work that Habitat for Humanity does and I want to be part of the excitement! As a donor, I will receive periodic updates on your construction activities but, more importantly, I know my gift will help a family in our community realize the dream of homeownership. **I would like to SHARE in your efforts against substandard housing in my community!** (Please print below)*

PLEASE SEND ME _____ SHARES at $54.17 EACH = $ $_____

In Honor Of: _____

Occasion: (Circle One)   HOLIDAY   BIRTHDAY   ANNIVERSARY

    OTHER: _____

Address of Recipient: _____

Gift From: _____   *Donor Address:* _____

Donor Email: _____

I AM ENCLOSING A CHECK FOR $ $_____ PAYABLE TO HABITAT FOR HUMANITY <u>OR</u> PLEASE CHARGE MY VISA OR MASTERCARD *(CIRCLE ONE)*

Card Number _____   Expiration Date: _____

Name as it appears on Credit Card _____   Charge Amount $ _____

Signature _____

Billing Address _____

Telephone # Day _____   Eve _____

PLEASE NOTE: Your contribution is tax-deductible to the fullest extent allowe~~d~~
Habitat for Humanity • P.O. Box 1443 • Newport News, VA 23601 • 75~~~~
www.HelpHabitatforHumanity.org

28.

CPSIA information can be obtained at www.ICGtesting.com
inted in the USA
OW011904220312

857BV00002B/7/P